The Diabetes
2-Month
Turnaround

LAURA HIERONYMUS, DNP, MLDE, BC-ADM, CDE

STACY GRIFFIN, PHARMD, LDE, CPT

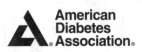

American
Diabetes
Association®

Director, Book Publishing, Abe Ogden; *Managing Editor,* Rebekah Renshaw; *Acquisitions Editor,* Victor Van Beuren; *Editor,* Andrea Braxton; *Production Manager,* Melissa Sprott; *Composition,* Circle Graphics; *Cover Design,* Jody Billert, Design Literate Studio; *Printer,* Versa Press.

Printed in the United States of America
1 3 5 7 9 10 8 6 4 2

The suggestions and information contained in this publication are generally consistent with the *Standards of Medical Care in Diabetes* and other policies of the American Diabetes Association, but they do not represent the policy or position of the Association or any of its boards or committees. Reasonable steps have been taken to ensure the accuracy of the information presented. However, the American Diabetes Association cannot ensure the safety or efficacy of any product or service described in this publication. Individuals are advised to consult a physician or other appropriate health care professional before undertaking any diet or exercise program or taking any medication referred to in this publication. Professionals must use and apply their own professional judgment, experience, and training and should not rely solely on the information contained in this publication before prescribing any diet, exercise, or medication. The American Diabetes Association—its officers, directors, employees, volunteers, and members—assumes no responsibility or liability for personal or other injury, loss, or damage that may result from the suggestions or information in this publication.

♾ The paper in this publication meets the requirements of the ANSI Standard Z39.48-1992 (permanence of paper).

ADA titles may be purchased for business or promotional use or for special sales. To purchase more than 50 copies of this book at a discount, or for custom editions of this book with your logo, contact the American Diabetes Association at the address below or at booksales@diabetes.org.

American Diabetes Association
2451 Crystal Drive, Suite 900
Arlington, VA 22202

DOI: 10.2337/9781580405669

Library of Congress Cataloging-in-Publication Data

Names: Hieronymus, Laura, author. | Griffin, Stacy, author.
Title: The diabetes 2-month turnaround / Laura Hieronymus, Stacy Griffin.
Description: Alexandria : American Diabetes Association, [2017] | Includes
  bibliographical references and index.
Identifiers: LCCN 2016032332 | ISBN 9781580405669 (paperback)
Subjects: LCSH: Diabetes—Popular works. | Diabetes—Treatment—Popular
  works. | Weight loss—Popular works. | Exercise—Popular works. | BISAC:
  HEALTH & FITNESS / Diseases / Diabetes. | HEALTH & FITNESS / Healthy
  Living. | HEALTH & FITNESS / Weight Loss. | HEALTH & FITNESS / Exercise.
Classification: LCC RC660.4 .H542 2017 | DDC 616.4/62406—dc23
LC record available at https://lccn.loc.gov/2016032332

Acknowledgments

To my husband, GD, whom I can always
count on, and our daughters,
Kelly and Lindsay—you are the most positive
and beautiful young women I know.
— LAURA —

To the people who have inspired me
throughout the years, including my mentor Laura,
my many colleagues, patients, and last,
but not least, my wonderful family.
— STACY —

To our friend, mentor, and colleague,
the late Patti Geil,
thank you for your supportive influence
and for teaching us to "carry on."
— LAURA & STACY —

Reviewers & Contributors

The authors would like to thank the reviewers for their careful reading of the manuscript and their insightful comments and suggestions.

Susan Braithwaite, MD

Martha Funnell, MS, RN, CDE

Tami A. Ross, RD, LD, MLDE, CDE

Sloane Mendelsohn, MS, RD
Associate Director, Nutrition, ADA

Jennifer Fassbender
Associate Director, Physical Fitness, ADA

Sheri Colberg-Ochs
Consultant, ADA

The authors would like to thank the following contributors to *8 Weeks to Maximizing Diabetes Control* (2008).

Christine Tobin, MBA, MSN, RN, CDE
Co-author of original version

John V. Borders, MD, FACP
Internal Medicine Specialist

Edward I. Galaid, MD, MPH
Internal Medicine/Preventive Medicine Specialist

Patti B. Geil, MS, RD, FADA, CDE
Diabetes Nutrition Educator

Kristina D. Humphries, MD
Endocrinology and Metabolism Specialist

Carol B. Peddicord, MD
Internal Medicine Specialist

Table of Contents

Foreword

While diabetes is one of the oldest diseases known to man, in the last 10 to 15 years the number of new type 2 diabetes diagnoses has far exceeded experts' predictions. Type 2 diabetes accounts for nearly 95% of all diabetes diagnoses, and while it was once known as "adult-onset" diabetes, it is now being diagnosed in a much younger population, including children and adolescents. Although it's encouraging that the amount of new diagnoses in the United States has begun to decline, the numbers are still very high. Nearly 28 million Americans are living with type 2 diabetes, and another 86 million have prediabetes, a serious health condition where blood glucose levels are higher than normal, but not high enough for a diabetes diagnosis. Prediabetes increases a person's risk of type 2 diabetes and other chronic diseases.

When type 2 diabetes isn't managed properly, it can lead to a higher risk for serious and often life-threatening complications. The triple threat of poorly managed diabetes, uncontrolled blood pressure, and abnormal cholesterol levels increases those individuals' risk for heart attacks and strokes as well as blindness, kidney failure, and nerve disease. But it doesn't have to be this way! Diabetes complications can be prevented! Medical research has shown that by taking an active role in managing your blood glucose levels, blood pressure, and cholesterol, you can potentially avoid these complications and live a full life.

Working closely with an interdisciplinary team of health-care professionals with expertise in medical care, nutrition, physical activity, pharmacy, and teaching self-care skills is the best way to manage your diabetes and prevent complications from arising. You are a key member of that diabetes care team.

The Diabetes 2-Month Turnaround combines current diabetes research with the authors' shared experience of more than 50 years as diabetes educators. This user-friendly book provides practical, comprehensive, step-by-step guidance along a two-month journey to better manage your diabetes. While written primarily for adults, many tips in this books may be applicable to younger individuals as well.

As a health-care professional committed to excellence in diabetes care, I encourage you to stay educated, maintain a positive outlook, and always keep the advice of your diabetes care team close to your heart.

— TAMI A. ROSS, RD, LD, MLDE, CDE

Type 2 Diabetes — Changing Your Behavior

Whether you've had type 2 diabetes for years or were recently diagnosed, you know that it is a life-changing disease. Even common activities, such as eating and exercising, are now much more complex because you have to worry about how they will affect your blood glucose levels. You might have been given instructions and suggestions about how to best manage your health, but you've probably found that some of this advice is easier said than done. Despite your efforts, you might not be seeing improvements to your health, or you might be feeling worse. This can indicate that you need to take a look at your self-care behaviors and try to make adjustments.

Understanding Type 2 Diabetes

Before you start taking steps to change how you manage your diabetes, it helps to understand the basics of the disease. Type 2 diabetes, the most common form of diabetes, occurs in nearly 95% of those diagnosed with the disease. It is estimated that of the 29.1 million Americans with diabetes, nearly 28 million have type 2 diabetes. Eight million of those people are unaware that they have it. With type 2 diabetes, the body usually produces insulin (the hormone that controls blood glucose) early on, but your body's muscle, fat, and liver cells have difficulty using the insulin properly. This is called "insulin resistance." Researchers believe that insulin resistance often occurs first in type 2 diabetes followed by a decline in pancreatic function and insulin production. As a result, the body has trouble metabolizing (breaking down) nutrients, primarily carbohydrate. Due to the lack of symptoms in some cases, type 2 diabetes may not be diagnosed until complications appear, which may be one reason why nearly one-third of the people living with the disease don't even know they have it. Type 2 diabetes is more common in those with one or more of the following risk factors:

- ▶ Being overweight or obese
- ▶ A lack of daily physical activity
- ▶ Use of tobacco products
- ▶ Older age (risk increases with aging)
- ▶ A first-degree relative (mother, father, or sibling) with type 2 diabetes
- ▶ A high-risk ethnicity (African American, Hispanic/Latino, American Indian, Asian American, or Pacific Islander)
- ▶ A history of prediabetes (blood glucose levels are higher than normal, but not high enough for a diabetes diagnosis)
- ▶ A history of gestational diabetes (diabetes that develops during pregnancy and ends upon delivery)
- ▶ Polycystic ovary syndrome (PCOS) (an endocrine disorder associated with insulin resistance)

- Acanthosis nigricans (a condition characterized by darkening of the skin folds of the armpits, neck, or groin; usually associated with obesity)
- High blood pressure
- A low HDL (good) cholesterol level and/or high triglyceride level (the storage form of fat in the body)
- A history of vascular problems (disease of the blood vessels)

Your Diabetes Care Team

There is nothing simple about dealing with this disease. The good news is that you can learn to self-manage your diabetes. It is essential that you work with your diabetes care team to make some healthful changes in behavior to help you optimally manage your blood glucose levels. Working with a team of diabetes care professionals has been shown to improve successful management of diabetes. Take an active role and collaborate with your team to gain insight into both your successes and struggles. Because you are the one who provides most of your diabetes care, you are ultimately the one in charge. You are the expert on you.

It's up to you to make sure the necessary members are part of your team. Typical team members include your primary care physician, registered nurse, and registered dietitian or registered dietitian nutritionist, but you can add as many people as you need. Each member has a specific role, but they should work together for a common goal—your diabetes health.

Medical Care
- Primary care physician (PCP)
- Endocrinologist (Endo)
- Advanced practice registered nurse (APRN), sometimes referred to as a "nurse practitioner"
- Physician assistant (PA)

Education and Support
- Licensed diabetes educator (LDE)
- Certified diabetes educator (CDE)

- ► Board certified - Advanced diabetes manager (BC-ADM)
- ► Registered dietitian (RD)/Registered dietitian nutritionist (RDN)
- ► Registered nurse (RN)
- ► Registered pharmacist (RPh or PharmD)
- ► Physical therapist (PT)
- ► Exercise physiologist (EP)
- ► Mental health professional (such as a psychologist or psychiatrist)

Medical Specialists

- ► Ophthalmologist/Optometrist (eye care)
- ► Podiatrist (toe and foot care)
- ► Nephrologist (kidney specialist)
- ► Neurologist (nerve specialist)
- ► Cardiologist (heart specialist)

Self-Care Behaviors

The Diabetes 2-Month Turnaround offers suggestions and guidance for adults with type 2 diabetes on a week-by-week basis. This eight-week structure puts into perspective diabetes self-management tasks and self-care behaviors that can seem overwhelming at times. The American Association of Diabetes Educators (AADE) developed an evidence-based framework of seven self-care behaviors that will help you and your diabetes care team measure, monitor, and manage your diabetes health outcomes. As you navigate life's ups and downs, it can be helpful to relate these seven self-care behaviors to your personal diabetes health.

This book discusses each behavior on a week-by-week basis. Let's start by becoming familiar with each of them:

Healthy Eating

Healthy eating is not a new concept. In fact, health-care professionals recommend healthy eating to the majority of their patients, not just those

AADE 7 SELF-CARE BEHAVIORS

Managing type 2 diabetes on a daily basis can be very challenging. To help you, diabetes educators have developed seven key areas to focus on. A diabetes educator can provide coaching and help you set priorities in these areas, so that you can live a healthy life.

1. Healthy Eating
2. Being Active
3. Monitoring
4. Taking Medication
5. Problem Solving
6. Reducing Risks
7. Healthy Coping

Adapted from: "AADE7 Self-Care Behaviors™," American Association of Diabetes Educators, accessed September 2016, https://www.diabeteseducator.org/patient-resources/ aade7-self-care-behaviors

with diabetes, because good nutrition is important for everyone. There isn't one set eating pattern that works for every person, so both you and the members of your care team should know how to apply healthy eating principles to your individualized meal plan.

Because what you eat affects your blood glucose levels, carefully considering each of your food choices is essential. These healthy eating goals can be applied to tracking your total carbohydrate amount, maintaining healthy portion sizes, and understanding the nutrition facts of the foods you eat.

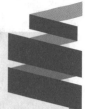

GOALS OF MEDICAL NUTRITION THERAPY

The American Diabetes Association (ADA) has identified four primary medical nutrition therapy (MNT) goals for adults with diabetes:

1. To promote and support healthful eating patterns, emphasizing a variety of nutrient-dense foods in appropriate portion sizes, in order to improve overall health and specifically to
   - Achieve and maintain body weight goals
   - Attain individualized glycemic, blood pressure, and lipid goals
   - Delay or prevent complications of diabetes
2. To address individual nutrition needs based on personal and cultural preferences, health literacy and numeracy, access to healthful foods, willingness and ability to make behavioral changes, and barriers to change
3. To maintain the pleasure of eating by providing nonjudgmental messages about food choices
4. To provide an individual with diabetes with practical tools for developing healthful eating patterns rather than focusing on individual macronutrients, micronutrients, or single foods

American Diabetes Association. Standards of Medical Care in Diabetes 2017. Diabetes Care *2017;40(Suppl.1):S34*

Being Active

Being active on a daily basis improves your overall physical health. Individuals who exercise regularly report increased self-esteem, reduced stress, and enhanced clarity of thought—who wouldn't want that? Routine physical activity also builds your confidence in your ability to make behavior changes. No matter what physical activity you choose to do, all of it counts toward better health.

The ADA recommends that adults with diabetes perform at least 150 minutes of moderate-intensity aerobic physical activity (rapid physical activity, such as walking, jogging, or swimming) a week. These 150 minutes should be spread over at least three days per week (preferably over five days a week), and you should try to go no more than two days in a row without exercise. Also, research shows that all individuals (not just those with diabetes) should reduce the amount of time they sit each day, so break up extended periods of sitting (longer than 30 minutes) by getting up and moving around. For people who do not have health complications that may make it unsafe to participate, resistance training—exercising with free weights or weight machines—is recommended at least twice weekly on nonconsecutive days. These exercises build muscle mass and help your body continue using glucose for energy between periods of exercise, which lowers your blood glucose levels.

For people with type 2 diabetes, it takes more insulin than normal to get glucose into the body's cells for energy. Exercise can improve muscle and liver sensitivity to insulin, which helps them use insulin better. Additional health benefits of physical activity include better weight management and decreased body fat, and when moderate-to-intense aerobic physical activity is done regularly, the risk for heart and blood vessel disease declines. Increased physical activity can also lead to lower total cholesterol levels, triglyceride levels, and blood pressure and to improved HDL (good) cholesterol levels, which is added protection against heart disease.

Monitoring

Monitoring is important because managing your blood glucose levels is essential for your health. When self-monitoring blood glucose (SMBG), recommended fasting levels for most non-pregnant adults with diabetes are 80 to 130 mg/dL and recommended levels for one to two hours after a meal are 180 mg/dL or less. Optimal blood glucose management is key to both feeling better on a day-to-day basis and lowering your risk for complications that can occur over time.

Managing your blood glucose takes a lot of work and commitment, but data suggest that by regularly monitoring your blood glucose levels, the better able you'll be to manage them. Routinely checking your blood glucose levels provides you and your diabetes care team with information to customize your treatment plan to best benefit your diabetes management.

To determine your overall improvement in blood glucose management, your diabetes care provider may also monitor your A1C measurement. The A1C is an index of average blood glucose for about 120 days, and the ADA's recommended A1C goal for most adults with diabetes is less than 7%. Lowered A1C levels are proof that you've improved your blood glucose management over the past two to three months.

Taking Medication

Taking medication to improve blood glucose management is generally recommended for individuals with type 2 diabetes. The goal is to develop a medication plan that will closely mimic the optimal use of insulin in the body. These medications, often used in combination, are prescribed to improve your health in one or more of the following ways:

- ▶ assist your pancreas to better release insulin
- ▶ help the body utilize insulin more efficiently
- ▶ help muscle, fat, and liver cells better respond to insulin
- ▶ reduce the amount of glucose in the bloodstream

The same diabetes medication may not be effective for everyone with the disease and your medication plan might need to change with your individual needs. Luckily, there are many choices and combinations of therapy, and the development of new and improved medications and new techniques for delivering medications every year may affect your medication regimen.

Problem Solving

Problem solving includes identifying the problem and developing a diabetes care plan to fix it. You will need to recognize and then respond to a number of situations, including blood glucose levels that are too high or too low and sick day management, which includes guidelines for dealing with an illness at home. Responding effectively to those issues as they present themselves will take both knowledge and skill. Therefore, to tackle any of the day-to-day problems of living with diabetes, you must first learn as much as you can about the disease.

Experts in your diabetes care team can help you learn more about diabetes and provide you with the tools for treating and preventing problems in the future. Your diabetes care plan is one such tool that is based on your diabetes care provider's recommendations but tailored to your individual lifestyle. The plan will become more refined as it evolves over time. With knowledge and experience and the help of your plan, you will find that you are more comfortable handling problems if they occur. Managing the ups and downs of blood glucose levels will require ongoing decisions about your food and activity choices and medication adjustments. While daily management of diabetes is up to you, you also have the expertise and support of your diabetes care team.

Reducing Risks

Reducing risks, both short term and long term, optimizes your diabetes health. Most long-term complications develop over 10 or more years, which may seem like a long time from now if you were recently diagnosed. However, because type 2 diabetes is typically not diagnosed until complications occur, your blood glucose level may have been too high for several years prior to your diagnosis.

Prevention is the best method to avoid serious problems with your diabetes. Learning about the possible complications is part of the diabetes care process, and many of these complications can be prevented or delayed by focusing on reducing risk factors. Managing blood glucose is an important aspect of preventive care because poorly managed blood glucose levels can lead to complications over time. The first goal of diabetes treatment after diagnosis is to eliminate the symptoms related to high blood glucose levels and to optimize blood glucose management in the short term. Long-term complications may be related to problems in the large blood vessels, such as heart disease and stroke, as well as issues in the small blood vessels and nerves, such as blindness, kidney failure, and nerve damage.

While diabetes is diagnosed based on the presence of hyperglycemia (high blood glucose), glucose management is not the only risk factor. High blood pressure and abnormal blood cholesterol and triglycerides will also lead to long-term complications. Preventing or detecting and then treating these complications ensures health and well-being. As you take charge of your diabetes, you will feel empowered, knowing that you are focusing on things that can make a difference in the long run.

Healthy Coping

Healthy coping with diabetes involves recognizing and responding appropriately to times when self-care behaviors feel challenging. Managing your diabetes requires around-the-clock responsibility, and you may feel angry, frightened, stressed, depressed, or overwhelmed, even to the point of denying that you have diabetes. These feelings are common when you consider how much of an impact diabetes has on your life.

Everyone encounters daily stressors, including family, work, school, deadlines, finances, or changes in physical and mental health. Stress can also occur from major life events, such as loss, divorce, changing jobs, moving, getting married, or the birth of a child. On top of those stressors that are common to most people, you have the added stressor of the long-term care of diabetes.

Healthy coping skills can eliminate or reduce the impact of these stressors. The key is understanding how your body reacts to stressors and then learning new ways to respond to stress. Although you need to actively participate in decision making, goal setting, and daily management, you are not expected to cope with your frustration and fears alone. This level of health management over time can be difficult, regardless of how motivated you are to live a long, healthy, and independent life. Expressing your feelings to your family, friends, and your diabetes care team is an essential step.

Taking Steps to Change

As you prepare to tackle these self-care behaviors, understand that mastering them takes time. Week 1 through Week 7 will focus on implementing the following 7 steps of personal behavior change:

- ► Knowledge
- ► Desire
- ► Skills
- ► Optimism
- ► Facilitation
- ► Stimulation
- ► Reinforcement

Week 8 will discuss maintaining changes for the future. Each chapter will provide an "action item" for each of the AADE7 self-care behaviors. The action items suggest steps that you can take that week toward improving your health, but you can use the format of this book as it best works for you.

To get started, you must recognize and understand why change is needed. This **knowledge**, along with learning all you can about diabetes, the importance of blood glucose management, and your treatment plan, is a first step in the right direction. Once you are equipped with the right knowledge, the **desire** (willingness) to make these changes is essential because knowing how to change is useless if you don't put it into practice. You can then begin to learn the **skills** associated with optimal blood glucose management. Do your best to stay **optimistic** because while taking care of yourself can be hard work sometimes, it's absolutely worth it. Your diabetes care team can help **facilitate** the learning process and help you take a primary role in managing your diabetes. Over time, hopefully the process will become easier, and once you see the benefits and impact of better blood glucose management on your short-term and long-term health, ideally you will be **stimulated**, or energized, to continue to make changes. Finally, focus on positive **reinforcement** by recognizing the changes you've made and by taking the time to reward yourself for a job well done!

Work with your diabetes care team to incorporate positive changes into your daily routine. It is also recommended that you track and record several different factors, including eating habits, blood glucose levels, and activity levels as well as your feelings, thoughts, and experiences as you work to improve your health. Keep this record with you, whether handwritten or on a computer or mobile device, because it will be useful to identify trends and to provide information to your diabetes care team. Finally, recognize that you won't be perfect and that adjustments will need to be made along the way. However, being willing to try is a great place to start.

WEEK 1

No Time Like the Present — Getting Started

Y ou have probably heard the phrase, "Knowledge is power." When it comes to diabetes, lifelong learning is crucial. The more you learn, the more insight you have. In fact, knowledge is one of your most important tools as you modify your behavior over time to best meet your needs. Don't forget to learn from your diabetes care team and from supplemental materials—like this book—that can also be helpful along the way. As significant new research in the area of diabetes is published and as more and more tools and technology become available, it always remains important for you to learn about the variety of evidence-based recommendations. Now, let's get started!

- ▶ **Healthy Eating:** Track your personal eating habits.
- ▶ **Being Active:** Learn about exercise safety.
- ▶ **Monitoring:** Check your meter for accuracy.
- ▶ **Take Medication:** Take inventory of your medications.
- ▶ **Problem Solving:** Learn how to manage hyperglycemia.
- ▶ **Reducing Risks:** Determine your target numbers.
- ▶ **Healthy Coping:** Find your motivation to live well with diabetes.

Healthy Eating: Your Personal Eating Habits

When trying to improve your healthy eating habits, the best place to start is by studying what you are eating now. Successful weight-loss programs ask participants to be accountable for what they eat, and the same concept applies to healthy eating even when weight loss isn't your goal. One way to be accountable is by keeping a record of foods eaten on a daily basis by writing the information down, using an online tool, or using a mobile application (app), such as MyFitnessPal or Fooducate. Then, review the records you've kept periodically to spot trends. To get started, include at least the following information as you track your food intake:

- ▶ Date
- ▶ Time you eat
- ▶ Reason for eating
- ▶ Food/drink consumed
- ▶ Total carbohydrate content
- ▶ Calorie intake

Along with the date, record the day of the week. Do you see any trends on certain days? For example, examine if and how your food intake changes based on how busy you are on a given day. As you record the food you are eating, take note of anything that surprises you. Perhaps you weren't aware that you consistently eat more on the weekends than during the week, for example. You can also record the different times that you eat during the day. Are you taking time for breakfast? How often are you eating on a daily basis? Again, look for anything that surprises you. You might not realize when and how often you are eating each day.

Adding comments about the reason you are eating any amount of food can help you determine what triggers your desire to eat. Start by asking yourself if you are hungry when you eat or if your eating is caused by some other factor. For example, do you sometimes eat because everyone else around you is eating? If so, how many servings are they eating and does that influence the amount that you choose to eat? You can also pay attention to how your mood and activities affect your eating habits. Do you eat when you feel nervous, bored, or depressed? Do you snack when you watch television or while you're on the computer?

Be specific about all of the types of food and drink you consume in one day. Don't just record that you ate a slice of bread, for example. Describe what kind of bread, whether that's white, whole wheat, whole grain, or honey wheat. Be as honest and accurate about the amount of food as possible by using a measuring cup and measuring spoons to determine the number of servings in a packaged food or drink. This level of specificity can help you and your registered dietitian (RD) or registered dietitian nutritionist (RDN) better evaluate the nutrition value of your choices.

Carbohydrate is the nutrient that most directly impacts your blood glucose levels. Therefore, it is helpful if you track carbohydrate content either in terms of the number of carbohydrate choices in a particular food (one choice = 15 grams of total carbohydrate) or simply the total number of grams of carbohydrate in the item consumed. You can usually find this information on a nutrition facts label. Tracking and recording carbohydrate can make you aware of the total carbohydrate content in the foods that you typically eat and help you determine if you are consistent with carbohydrate from meal to meal.

Through monitoring, you may find that some of your favorite foods are higher in calories than you suspected. While you don't have to totally give up these foods, perhaps you can eat them less frequently or in smaller amounts. By taking some steps to modify a recipe, such as using a low-fat alternative to a recipe ingredient, you can lower the fat and calorie amounts without sacrificing the good taste. When you compare your calories day to day, you can notice patterns to help you make decisions to lessen overall calorie consumption and provide better consistency in caloric amounts on a daily basis. You may also find that by tracking calories, you become more aware of the nutrition content and portion size of the foods you are eating.

Record keeping can be a valuable tool for learning about your eating habits. Be sure to periodically share food records with members of your diabetes care team, especially your RD/RDN, to assure you are staying on track and to develop strategies to make healthier choices.

Being Active: Exercise Safety

Choosing an exercise routine that works for you means first knowing what your body can handle. It is important that you discuss any significant change in your activity levels with your diabetes care provider during your regular office visits. In some cases, there may be limitations or restrictions to your exercise plan or a better activity to choose from. Not all activities are right for everyone with diabetes. Be careful when starting new activities, and check with your diabetes care provider if you have questions.

If necessary, formal exercise testing can help identify the presence of underlying heart and blood vessel problems. If you are relatively healthy and are planning a moderate-intensity activity like walking, testing is usually not required or recommended. If you have diabetes-related complications, your provider can make some suggestions about the type of exercise that is best for you, and in the case of hyperglycemia, he or she may recommend that you delay exercise until your levels are closer to your recommended range. This suggestion mainly applies to people who have ketones (chemical compounds produced when fats are used for energy instead of glucose). Without ketones, simply use caution when starting out with elevated blood glucose levels and only exercise when you feel well. Be sure to stay hydrated during the activity.

Exercise and Hypoglycemia

Blood glucose management can be enhanced with regular physical activity; however, be on the lookout for symptoms of hypoglycemia (blood glucose levels that are too low). Hypoglycemia is not as common during physical activity for people with type 2 diabetes as it is for those with type 1. However, you are at an increased risk for hypoglycemia if you are taking certain blood glucose–lowering medications, specifically insulin and/or oral insulin secretagogues (medications that cause the pancreas to secrete more insulin).

Usually your diabetes care team will recommend that you delay exercise if your blood glucose levels are outside of recommended ranges prior to exercise. The effect of exercise on your blood glucose level depends on many factors, including the time of day you plan to exercise, how often and intensely you exercise, the timing of your diabetes medicines, and when and what you ate. If you plan to exercise moderately or vigorously for 45 minutes or more, make sure to carry carbohydrates with you that you can use to treat hypoglycemia if it should occur and to keep blood glucose levels balanced. Although most people won't need one, it is possible that you could also need a carbohydrate snack if you are unable to adjust your medication that can cause hypoglycemia.

Monitoring: Meter Accuracy

If you have been monitoring your blood glucose levels, keep it up! If you haven't, there is no time like the present to get started. Not all blood glucose measuring devices (meters) are equal, so it is important to talk with a diabetes educator about your meter choices. First off, make sure your blood glucose meter is in working order and that your test strips are up to date. If your strips are unopened, they are good until the manufacturer expiration date stamped on the bottle or box. If they have been opened, then they are usually good for about two to three months, but you can check the package insert in the test strip box to verify how long the opened strips are recommended for use. Using the opened test strips after the recommended date can lead to inaccurate results when checking your blood glucose.

If your meter is more than a couple of years old, ask a member of your diabetes care team about an update. Many times that person will have sample meters that are newer versions of the meter you are currently using, and these updated versions may still work with your current test strips. You can also call the company that manufactures your meter to see what updated options are currently available. You might have better access to the appropriate supplies if you use the most current versions of self-monitoring equipment. If you have insurance, ask about the coverage for an updated model. You will likely need a prescription to obtain insurance coverage for the blood glucose meter and supplies.

Each company typically lists a toll-free number on the back of the meter. You can call that number to learn how to get a glucose control solution for the meter. The solution contains a controlled amount of glucose that, when applied correctly, should read within a certain designated range printed on the test strip packaging. It can be used to verify that the meter is reading test strips correctly. If you already have glucose control solution, check to make sure that it isn't past the expiration date that is printed on the bottle. If you've opened it before, verify that it is not past the discard date, which is usually the date opened plus about three months. That way you can be sure that you're getting accurate results when you test. It is a good idea to check your blood glucose meter with a control solution as recommended by the manufacturer. Follow these steps to perform a control test:

1. Shake the bottle and apply a drop of solution to the test strip (or follow the steps recommended by the manufacturer's user guide).
2. The meter will read the solution on the strip similar to reading a blood sample.
3. If the result of your control solution test is not within the specified range printed on the packaging, repeat the test to verify.
4. If it is still not within the recommended range, call the meter company and ask about getting a replacement.

Alternate Site Testing

Some people don't like sticking their fingers. While fingertips have traditionally been used for sampling blood glucose, some meters work with blood samples from other sites, including the arm, thigh, or palm. If alternative site testing is important to you, discuss this with your diabetes care team and be sure that the meter you have, or one that you might purchase, is approved for such testing.

Not all meters are approved for the same sites and some sites may not be right for you, but these meters can usually be used with the fingertips in addition to the alternative site. Be sure you are instructed in the proper use of the meter because the procedure and equipment may be different for the alternative site. However, it is generally best to use the fingertips when rapid blood glucose changes are likely to occur, like when you have recently exercised, recently taken insulin, or eaten within the last two hours. Blood flow reaches the finger or palm at the base of the thumb three to five times faster than alternate sites, so fingertip samples may show these rapid changes sooner than other areas.

Taking Medication: Medication Inventory

Taking your medications helps you avoid the short-term complications of diabetes and prevent or delay the long-term complications. Chances are you already have a full medicine cabinet. You may take oral medications prescribed for diabetes, blood pressure, and cholesterol, and you may be taking an injectable diabetes medication as well. On top of that, you might need over-the-counter (OTC) medications, such as vitamins, pain relievers, heartburn medications, cold medicines, allergy medications, and herbal supplements.

While taking a variety of medications can mean more health benefits, it also means more potential risks. However, there are steps you can take to increase the benefits and reduce the risks. Once you commit to focusing on your medications, it will take some organization and time. Begin by gathering all of your prescription and OTC medications. Next, make an up-to-date list of these medications. Your pharmacist should be able to print a complete list of all your prescriptions. Record the name of the medication, the dosage, the reason you are taking the medication, and the time(s) of day you take it. Keeping the list on a computer or tablet can help you avoid having to rewrite the list each time an update is necessary. Remember to add the new date when you update the list and keep your medication list with you in case of questions from your care team.

If you already have a list of all of your medications, be sure your list stays updated. This can also help with "spring cleaning" for your medicine cabinet, which involves disposing of expired medications, medications that have been discontinued or are no longer safe, or medications that you no longer use.

Prescription medications usually have a "medication guide," and the label that is on the bottle or package also provides information on how to take your medicine. Your pharmacy may also provide drug information on printed forms when you pick up your prescriptions. Don't forget to also check the labels and package inserts (if available) on your OTC items. Always read any information that comes with your medications as it contains answers to many questions you may have.

The Federal Drug Administration (FDA) estimates that 50% of people do not take their prescriptions correctly, which causes medications to work less effectively. This risk of taking your medication incorrectly increases if you take many different medications. All of these can cause side effects if taken improperly. It is a good idea to check with your diabetes care team or pharmacist before taking any OTC medications or herbal supplements in case of potential interactions with your current medicines. Be sure you have all the facts about all of your medications, including the possible results of not following through with your doctor's medication recommendations. Ask yourself these important questions:

► What is the name of this medication?
► Does my health-care team know I take it?
► Why am I taking it?

- How much should I take?
- What time of day should I take it?
- How should I take it (with or without food)?
- How often do I use this medication (daily, every other day, weekly)?
- What problems (if any) do I have taking it?
- Are there any potential interactions (a change in the effects of a medication because it reacts with another medication, with foods or beverages, or with a preexisting medical condition) or side effects?
- What is the expiration date?
- How many refills do I have left?

Many of these answers can be found on the packaging of the medication or in the package insert. If you can't find the answer, write down the question and have it ready for your next visit with your diabetes care provider. You can also discuss your questions with your pharmacist. Keeping an updated list makes it easier to recall the medications you are taking, particularly if you are meeting with several different diabetes care providers. Store all important medication information in a location that works for you, such as a drawer in your bedroom.

Ask your diabetes care team if you have a "patient portal" option that you can use to list and track your medications. In the past few years, the federal government has created incentives for health-care institutions to put patient portals in place to ensure consumers have electronic access to their protected health information (PHI). A patient portal is a secure online tool provided through a health-care system that allows you to retrieve your PHI online anytime, anywhere. Most portals allow you to see information from your recent health-care visits as well as a current list of medications, lab values, any allergies you have, and immunizations. This resource has a number of health benefits, and while components of patient portals may vary, a key feature is that the information is secure and protected.

Problem Solving: Hyperglycemia

When self-monitoring your blood glucose, recommended fasting levels for most non-pregnant adults with diabetes are 80 to 130 mg/dL, and recommended blood glucose levels 1 to 2 hours after a meal are 180 mg/dL or less. When your levels are higher than these ranges, it is called hyperglycemia, which is a factor in the development of long-term complications. The cause of high blood glucose can involve one or several factors, but these are the most common reasons:

- ▶ Forgetting to take your diabetes medications
- ▶ Not taking enough diabetes medication
- ▶ A change in diabetes medication
- ▶ Overeating
- ▶ Not exercising enough or regularly
- ▶ Another medical condition, such as an infection or the flu

To resolve this problem, start by asking your health-care provider for your individual target numbers for blood glucose if you do not already know your target range (Week 1, Reducing Risks, page 24). Recognizing and responding to the symptoms of hyperglycemia promptly, especially those you commonly experience, will also enable you to reduce or avoid complications.

If you don't have an infection, getting back to the basics (a balance of medications, meal planning, and physical activity) can often lower your blood glucose back within your target range. If blood glucose continues to climb to levels above 240 mg/dL, call your health-care provider. Report your symptoms, what you have eaten, and the medications you have taken, including the name, dose, and timing. Also, make sure your hands are clean prior to performing a blood glucose test to assure there is nothing on the site that could affect the accuracy of your test. Look at your medications to see if they have changed in color or appearance, indicating they have lost potency or expired.

HYPERGLYCEMIA SYMPTOMS AND TREATMENTS

Symptoms
- ▶ Excessive thirst or hunger
- ▶ Frequent urination, especially at night
- ▶ A tired or sleepy feeling
- ▶ Lack of energy
- ▶ Blurred vision
- ▶ Frequent infections
- ▶ Slow healing of cuts or sores
- ▶ Dry or itchy skin

Treatments
- ▶ Check and record your blood glucose more frequently, and look for patterns of hyperglycemia.
- ▶ Take your correct dose of medication as recommended.
- ▶ Ask your health-care team about increasing or changing your medication.
- ▶ Follow your meal plan.
- ▶ Make adjustments to your current meal plan, such as eating less.
- ▶ Increase your physical activity.

Prolonged Hyperglycemia

Prolonged hyperglycemia can lead to diabetic ketoacidosis (DKA) or hyperosmolar hyperglycemic state (HHS). DKA is a combination of severe hyperglycemia, dehydration, acidosis (increased acidity in blood or tissue), and ketosis (a buildup of ketones in the body). It occurs when there is a severe deficiency of insulin in the body, and blood glucose levels can reach levels of over 600 mg/dL. Those with type 2 diabetes may develop ketoacidosis when they have acute infections or trauma that place their bodies under great physical stress. Respiratory tract infections like the flu or pneumonia and gastroenteritis (stomach bug) are common causes of DKA, so special care is necessary when you are experiencing an illness. Symptoms include nausea, vomiting, very dry mouth, extreme tiredness, shortness of breath, and dehydration. HHS is a combination of hyper-glycemia and dehydration, much like DKA, but without the presence of ketones. Prompt medical attention is essential to treat both of these serious conditions because they may lead to a change in mental state, loss of consciousness, and possibly death.

Prevention of hyperglycemia, as well as DKA or HHS, begins with diabetes self-management education on how to recognize the symptoms and take action. If your blood glucose is greater than 240 mg/dL, you may want to check your urine for ketones. Without insulin, your body cannot use glucose in your bloodstream for energy, so ketones are chemical com-pounds produced when fats are used for energy instead of glucose. They become dangerous when they build to extremely high levels in the blood. You can get ketone test strips at your pharmacy and use them to test your urine. If you have elevated blood glucose levels and your urine is positive for ketones, call your physician immediately.

Reducing Risks: Target Goals

To successfully reduce your risk of complications, you must clearly under-stand your target goals not only for blood glucose, but for blood pressure and lipid levels as well. Your target goals are individualized numbers determined by your diabetes care providers to keep you in optimal health. If you are unsure of your target goals, ask a member of your diabetes care team at your next appointment.

The ADA Standards of Care make target goal recommendations for adults with diabetes. These targets are based on clinical research that determines the numbers that decrease your risk of complications. Over time, as newer research is available, the recommendations may be

ADA RECOMMENDATIONS

Blood glucose
- ▶ A1C of less than 7%
- ▶ A fasting glucose of 80 to 130 mg/dL
- ▶ A 1- to 2-hour post-meal glucose of less than 180 mg/dL

Blood pressure
- ▶ Blood pressure of less than 140/90 mmHg

Lipids
- ▶ LDL (bad) cholesterol of less than 100 mg/dL
- ▶ HDL (good) cholesterol greater than 40 mg/dL in men and 50 mg/dL in women
- ▶ Triglyceride levels of less than 150 mg/dL

modified. Therefore, it is important to have ongoing discussions regarding these target goals with your diabetes care team and to stay aware of any changes in recommendations.

Your health-care provider can give you an assessment and monitor your risks for developing complications. Always ask for a copy of your lab values, and if you have access to a patient portal through your diabetes care provider, you will likely be able to obtain your lab results there. By keeping track of your lab results, you can compare them to the ADA target goals and to the goals set with your diabetes care team. Use this information to discuss treatment options with your team. For example, "statins" are the therapy of choice for lipid management. Lipids are fats in the body that are usually broken down and used for energy, and a statin is an oral medication that inhibits an enzyme that plays a role in the body's production of cholesterol. Statins have been found to reduce heart disease and mortality (death rate) in those who are at risk. The intensity of statin therapy (medication and dose) recommended will vary based upon your age and the presence of other risk factors. They are recommended for all people with diabetes who are 40 or older, and people with diabetes under 40 may also be recommended to take statins if they have additional heart and blood vessel risk factors. Other therapies may be prescribed in addition to a statin if HDL or triglycerides are outside of the recommended targets.

Healthy Coping: Living Well with Diabetes

Living with diabetes can create strong feelings such as uncertainty, frustration, resentment, or anger. Many feel they have no control of their lives or that the recommended self-care behaviors are too difficult. Look for ways to fit diabetes self-care behaviors into your current lifestyle. Explore methods that you can use every day, such as talking with a supportive friend or family member, meditating or praying, or seeking the support of a member of your health-care team.

Learn as much as you can about diabetes, but remember that it is a lifelong process. Don't expect to do it all at once. Know what works for you and what you are able and willing to do to manage your diabetes. You have made and will make many decisions about your meal plan, activity levels, and medications. This experience and knowledge will help you make lifestyle changes today and in the future.

To live well with diabetes, you need both motivation and resilience. Motivation is an incentive that moves you to action. Perhaps you're motivated to exercise because you feel better afterward or perhaps you're motivated to keep a record of your blood glucose levels because you're searching for patterns. Think about things that have motivated you in the past, whether they were related to diabetes or not, and consider how they can continue to motivate you. Resiliency is your ability to recover quickly from illness, misfortune, or other types of negative changes. We have all met or heard of people who have overcome insurmountable odds, such as veterans, activists, entrepreneurs, athletes, or even friends and family. Consider what you can learn from them and others to find your own personal strengths. You've probably shown resiliency in the past as well. Maybe it was during a health or financial challenge, a surprising change in your life, or the loss of someone special to you. What inspired you to keep going during those situations? Figuring this out will take some thought, and you might want to record your conclusions for future reference. Discover what makes you strong and keeps you motivated and use it to achieve the long-term results you want.

Perfect diabetes self-care is impossible, so you haven't failed if you are having trouble with a certain part of your care. Instead of beating yourself up, think about ways that you can make adjustments. Negative self-talk can be very destructive, so focus on what you are doing well. Understanding and cooperation with medical recommendations can also enhance a sense of well-being. And by all means, congratulate or reward yourself for your efforts along the way.

WEEK 2

Diabetes Self-Management — Set Goals

Y ou have to have the desire and motivation to successfully make changes in your behavior. Think about why it is important for you to maintain your diabetes health. These reasons might include: reducing the risk of complications or simply feeling better on a daily basis. Once you have determined the "whys" for taking care of yourself, then start doing. For example, meeting with an RD/RDN to learn about healthy eating gets you on the right track because you can develop a healthful meal plan, which is a useful tool. However, just having the tool won't be enough until you actually use it. Your motivation has to be strong enough that the long-term payoff of making a difficult change is better than the short-term satisfaction of continuing your current behaviors. So, what

- ▶ **Healthy Eating:** Plan your target total carbohydrate amounts.
- ▶ **Being Active:** Develop an exercise routine.
- ▶ **Monitoring:** Check and track your blood glucose.
- ▶ **Taking Medication:** Learn your medication side effects and interactions.
- ▶ **Problem Solving:** Learn how to manage hypoglycemia.
- ▶ **Reducing Risks:** Make a plan to reach your target numbers.
- ▶ **Healthy Coping:** Empower yourself through personal goals.

is it that you really want? For example, do you want to eat healthier to optimize your blood glucose management and improve your chances of living a long and healthy life? Think about your long-term goals, your priorities, and the importance of diabetes health in getting there.

Healthy Eating: Total Carbohydrate Amounts

As you continue to track your eating habits, pay close attention to the total carbohydrate content in the foods you eat. Carbohydrate is the nutrient that most directly influences blood glucose levels after eating. Work with your health-care provider to determine the healthiest amount of carbohydrate grams for each meal and snack that you eat and set goals based on these amounts. The two of you will consider your age, activity level, any other medical issues you might have, as well as any weight-loss goals.

If you are on a set diabetes medication schedule, it is usually recommended that you keep carbohydrate consistent throughout the day to help steady blood glucose levels. In this case, it is best to try and stay as close as possible to the number of grams of total carbohydrate recommended for meals and snacks. If you take insulin at mealtime (either by injection or insulin pump), you may need to adjust your mealtime insulin based on the amount of carbohydrate you eat each meal. Spreading carbohydrate out through the day can help minimize the glucose load in your body at any given time. Snacks can also help steady your levels as well as prevent hunger between meals.

Until you see your health-care provider, set a target goal to maintain as consistent of a carbohydrate intake as possible. If you have questions, keep notes so your care provider can help you better understand your meal planning efforts. Just as you would follow up with your physician if he or she prescribed a medication for you, be sure to do the same if you're seeing an RD/RDN. Follow-up visits can help you adjust your carbohydrate and nutrition needs to help you get the best possible glucose management.

Being Active: Your Exercise Routine

Once you've received any necessary medical clearance and have had any questions about physical activity answered, you are ready to start. Think about your daily routine and about how you might add activity into your everyday life. Look at what you do during the week that includes walking or other physical activities and come up with different ways to increase your efforts. Maybe you always watch TV after coming home from work; could you exercise as you watch? Maybe you walk your dog every day; could you walk at a faster pace or walk for a longer distance?

Many people find that an activity tracker is helpful in determining the distance walked on a daily basis. Basic models may be purchased for as little as $10 to $25, while high-tech versions can cost significantly more. There are also mobile apps that you can use if you carry your smartphone with you throughout the day, and many apps can sync with fitness trackers to provide you with even more information. Because trackers sense movement, they may not be good at making fine measurements; movement as simple as shifting in your chair can be picked up by the tracker. However, some trackers take this into account and don't begin counting until you have taken repeated steps to ensure that the movement is repetitive. While trackers often can't give you precise measurements, they can give you a general idea of what you are doing during the day.

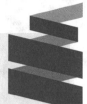

TAKE SMALL STEPS FOR GETTING MORE PHYSICAL ACTIVITY

► **Dress to move:** Shoes should be supportive with thick, flexible soles to cushion steps. Wear dry, comfortable clothing and socks.

► **Start slowly:** Begin with a 5-minute walk or other activity on most days each week and slowly build up to 30 minutes 5 days a week.

► **Build physical activity into your day:** Walk the dog, park the car farther from the entrance, and add activities such as leg lifts or walking in place during a TV show.

► **Move more at work:** Walk during breaks or lunch, take the stairs instead of the elevator, stand and walk during phone calls, or switch to a standing desk or treadmill desk.

► **Count your steps/minutes:** Use an activity tracker, such as a pedometer, accelerometer, or a mobile app, to track your number of steps or minutes of physical activity each day.

► **Stretch:** Perform stretches before and after activity to avoid stiff muscles. Stretch only as far as is comfortable, and make sure you warm your muscles up before stretching with some light activity.

► **Make it social:** Walk with family and friends. Add physical activity, such as soccer, hiking, or bowling, to social events.

► **Have fun:** Dance to your favorite music, play a sport, or do another activity that is fun but also gets you moving. Change up your physical activities so you won't get bored.

► **Keep it up:** The longer you keep up your exercise routine, the better you will feel and the more likely you are to keep going.

Adapted from: "Small Steps. Big Rewards. Your GAME PLAN to Prevent Type 2 Diabetes: Information for Patients," *National Institutes of Health, accessed October 2016, http://www.niddk.nih.gov/health-information/health-communication-programs/ndep/ health-care-professionals/game-plan/small-steps*

Two methods to monitor your physical activity are tracking your number of steps taken or your number of minutes of activity on a daily basis. Walking 2,000 steps per day is an approximate equivalent to walking one mile for most adults. This will take the average adult about 17 to 22 minutes, but can vary based on fitness level. The ADA recommends walking 30 minutes a day, five days a week. If you are not used to walking, build up gradually as your fitness improves:

1. Track the number of steps or minutes you are walking on a daily basis for one week. As a reference point, walking 10,000 steps per day is an approximate equivalent to walking five miles for most adults.
2. At the end of the week, take the highest number of steps or minutes that you recorded on a given day and use that as your starting baseline for the next week.
3. If this number is comfortable for you, add 500 steps (approximately a quarter of a mile) or about five minutes per day the following week.
4. Keep increasing until you reach your goal.

Whether you are tracking steps or minutes, avoid going more than two days per week without exercise or your insulin action will start to decrease. You'll benefit the most by spreading the physical activity effort out over the week. While walking outside is usually preferred by most, indoor alternatives such as mall walking, watching exercise videos on a DVD or online, or using a treadmill or exercise bike are great options to help you stay on track during bad weather.

Monitoring: When to Check Blood Glucose

Once you make sure that your meter is accurate, the information that you gather from self-monitoring of blood glucose will be useful to you and your diabetes care team. Ask your diabetes care team to help you determine the times of day to monitor. Depending on the amount of test strips available to you based on your insurance plan, you may have to check your blood glucose at different times each day, but you can also check your blood levels whenever you feel it is necessary. Monitoring can help you determine how well your diabetes treatment plan is working. Common times that are recommended include:

- ▶ Fasting (pre-breakfast)
- ▶ Before meals
- ▶ After meals
- ▶ Before bedtime
- ▶ In the middle of the night

Pre-meal blood glucose checks are probably the most commonly recommended checks. This includes the pre-breakfast check, which will most likely be your fasting check when you first wake up (after 8 to 12 hours of no food intake). Pre-meal checks provide information about your overall diabetes treatment plan because your levels aren't affected by food or drink you've consumed.

In some cases, after-meal blood glucose readings can help you assess the impact of food choices, the amount of food, and carbohydrate intake on blood glucose management. Your diabetes care team might recommend checking approximately one to two hours after you begin eating. This result is probably most useful if you check before the meal and compare that with the post-meal result. The after-meal value can also assist you and your diabetes care team in evaluating the effect of diabetes medications that are taken to manage post-meal blood glucose. If you have pre-meal blood glucose values within your target ranges, yet your A1C remains above target, then monitoring post-meal values with diabetes care intervention(s) to reduce post-meal blood glucose may improve your A1C.

Occasional bedtime checks may be recommended to determine if your blood glucose level is safe prior to going to sleep. Bedtime checks compared to fasting blood glucose checks the following morning can verify the effects of your treatment plan overnight. They may also help you to determine if you need a bedtime snack.

Checking your blood glucose level in the middle of the night is particularly useful to insulin users to determine if blood glucose levels are maintained at a reasonably safe level during the night. In some cases, if fasting or pre-breakfast levels are too high, it can be the result of rebounding from glucose levels that have dropped too low during the night. If you or your diabetes care team decide that you need to do a middle of the night check, your team will usually recommend taking a reading sometime between 2 and 4 a.m. This is especially true for those taking intermediate or long-acting insulin therapy injected at supper or bedtime and is also useful for evaluating pre-programmed overnight basal rates if you are using an insulin pump.

Besides those regular times, it is important to check your blood glucose level to verify feelings and symptoms of hyperglycemia and hypoglycemia. It is important to establish a plan ahead of time with your diabetes care team to promptly treat these hyperglycemia or hypoglycemia events. Monitoring can also be useful when evaluating the effects of physical activity on blood glucose management, so you may want to check both before and after an activity. Be sure to check your blood glucose before driving or operating machinery because these situations can be dangerous if hypoglycemia should occur.

Be sure to record your blood glucose levels whenever you check them. Make sure to include the day and time, blood glucose result, any medication taken, and any adjustments made, as well as what you ate (or if you ate anything different than usual) and any exercise you participated in. Many meters have the option of downloading the results with company-based software. To find out more about this option, ask your diabetes care team or call the toll-free number on the back of your meter. Take the record with you when you visit your health-care providers, and always take your meter with you to your appointments as many diabetes care providers will download the meter results at their office. This allows you and your diabetes care team to promptly discuss your patterns of blood glucose readings. Regardless of the method you choose for tracking your blood glucose results, the important thing is that you have information to help you and your diabetes team make decisions about your care.

Keeping Track of Your Blood Glucose Numbers

Record keeping can help you determine patterns and whether or not you are meeting your goals. By checking at least once daily and alternating your times, you can see how you are doing at various times of day. When you look at the blood glucose record below, what do you see? What is the pattern before breakfast, lunch, and dinner? Identifying patterns helps you figure out how well your plan is working and is useful to determine any needed adjustments.

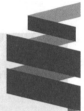

WEEKLY DIABETES RECORD

Week Starting _____ (include date range)

	Mon	Tues	Wed	Thurs	Fri	Sat	Sun
Other Blood Glucose							
Breakfast Blood Glucose	156 mg/dL			139 mg/dL			154 mg/dL
Medicine							
Lunch Blood Glucose		185 mg/dL			155 mg/dL		
Medicine							
Dinner Blood Glucose			90 mg/dL			85 mg/dL	
Medicine							
Bedtime Blood Glucose							
Medicine							
Notes (Special events, sick days, exercise)							

This chart is an example only and in no way reflects personal goals.

Taking Medication: Medication Side Effects and Interactions

As you are prescribed new medications, be sure to ask about side effects and when you should report the effects of a new medication to your diabetes care team. If you start any new medication and find your blood glucose is higher or lower, check with your care team to make sure it is not due to your new medication.

Here are some general tips to manage your medication side effects and interactions:

▶ Choose a pharmacy where a pharmacist is available to answer questions and will take an interest in your medical needs. Consult with your pharmacist about any medication changes as well as for an annual medication review.

▶ Get as many of your prescriptions filled at the same pharmacy as possible, and keep your allergy information up to date. The pharmacist will be able to check your prescriptions, keeping your allergy history in mind, and will look for any potential interactions with other medications that you take.

▶ Understand the benefits and risks of your prescriptions. Your pharmacist should tell you if there are any side effects associated with medications that you are prescribed.

▶ If you are considering taking an OTC medication, check with your pharmacist. He or she will be able to look at other medications that you are taking to see if there are concerns before making a recommendation.

▶ Save the pharmacy printouts and place them with your medical records. You may want to consider keeping a folder that includes this information.

Side effects are sometimes related to mistakenly taking an extra dose of a medication. Using one pharmacy for all your prescriptions can help you avoid medication errors by preventing duplicate medications or interactions. The pharmacy can also alert you if a medication has been ordered that could cause an allergic reaction.

One of the most common side effects of medications that increase insulin in the bloodstream, such as oral insulin secretagogues or insulin injections, is the risk of hypoglycemia. You may experience hypoglycemia if lifestyle factors like physical activity, food intake, or alcohol consumption are out of balance with your medications. Hypoglycemia is easily treated with 15 to 20 grams of carbohydrate (ideally a glucose source, such as glucose tablets or glucose gel), which should start working quickly. Some diabetes medications do not have a risk for hypoglycemia when taken alone; however, the risk increases when they are added to oral insulin secretagogues or insulin. It is important to understand how each of your medications works in the body to determine if you are at risk for hypoglycemia. If you have a question about this, ask a member of your diabetes care team.

Some medications taken to reduce high blood pressure can raise blood glucose levels. If you take blood pressure medications and your blood glucose levels increase, it may be due to a medication interaction. Medications used for other purposes, such as improving lipid levels, can also raise blood glucose, while other medications can make oral diabetes medications more potent, which may lower blood glucose.

Some diabetes medications may cause side effects of nausea, gas, bloating, or diarrhea. This might occur when you first take the medications and may decrease or disappear over time. If you believe you are having side effects from your medications, be sure to tell your diabetes care provider. Your diabetes care team can work with you to minimize the discomfort while maximizing the effectiveness of your medications.

For some medications, your doctor will start you on a low dose and gradually increase the dose as needed. This is called "titration" and should help ease some of the side effects by allowing your body to gradually get used to the medication. For example, the oral medication metformin may be titrated over weeks to minimize adverse events. It is important to allow enough time for the medication to have its full therapeutic effect. Your body may need time to adjust to a new medication, so ask how long you should wait before calling to report symptoms. If the side effect is unbearable, call your health-care provider. If you stop taking a medication because of the side effects, try to talk to your diabetes care team as soon as possible to make adjustments to your treatment. There are many other medication options available, so speak up.

Problem Solving: Hypoglycemia

Hypoglycemia is the result of elevated amounts of insulin that lower blood glucose to levels that are less than desirable. It can be conservatively defined as blood glucose levels of 70 mg/dL or less with symptoms. Significant hypoglycemia is considered to be a blood glucose level of less than 54 mg/dL. Keep in mind, certain individuals experience symptoms at different levels. How long you've had diabetes may play a role in whether you will feel symptoms or not. People who have had diabetes for a long time may not even recognize that they are experiencing low blood glucose symptoms. In some cases, people are unable to recognize hypoglycemia in the early stages, which is called "hypoglycemia unawareness." This can prevent a person from getting treatment in a timely manner, especially if a person's symptoms impair his or her ability to treat the hypoglycemia. People with hypoglycemia unawareness, those who are elderly or live alone, as well as young children are often given higher target blood glucose goals for treating hypoglycemia for safety reasons. Lower target numbers for treatment of hypoglycemia may be recommended in pregnant women with diabetes.

There are several factors that can increase the risk for hypoglycemia in type 2 diabetes, including advancing age, poor nutritional status, and hepatic (liver) or renal (diabetic kidney) disease. Hypoglycemia can also occur if you take too much of certain medications, exercise too long, eat too little, or consume too much alcohol. Anyone who takes oral insulin secretagogues or insulin can have low blood glucose reactions, and even if a medication has a low risk for hypoglycemia, when added to an oral insulin secretagogue or insulin, the risk for hypoglycemia may increase once blood glucose management improves.

Initial symptoms of hypoglycemia are caused by hormones that are released by the body to help increase blood glucose levels. These warning signs of hypoglycemia are weakness, shakiness, sweatiness or clamminess, rapid heart rate, and hunger. If levels continue to drop, the brain suffers from a lack of glucose. Low blood glucose reactions are categorized as mild or severe, and the majority of hypoglycemic cases for people with type 2 diabetes are mild reactions. A mild reaction results in symptoms like:

- ► Sweating
- ► Trembling
- ► Lightheadedness
- ► Difficulty concentrating
- ► Changes in vision
- ► Slurred speech
- ► Loss of coordination
- ► Headaches
- ► Dizziness
- ► Drowsiness
- ► Mood changes (nervousness, being argumentative or aggressive, crying)

Usually, mild symptoms can be quickly identified and treated by drinking or eating carbohydrate. A severe reaction occurs when people are unable to treat themselves because of confusion or unconsciousness. In some cases, seizures and death can result from severe hypoglycemia. Because of the inability to self-treat a severe reaction, others must administer the treatment to raise your blood glucose levels. Glucagon is an injectable medication that is available by prescription only. Close friends and family members should know where it is stored and when and how to administer.

TREATMENT FOR HYPOGLYCEMIA

To treat hypoglycemia, first use your meter to check your blood glucose to confirm. If your blood glucose is below your target level, treat it promptly. Pure glucose is the preferred treatment, but any form of carbohydrate that converts to glucose will increase the blood glucose level.

Preferred pure glucose sources:
- ▶ 3 to 5 glucose tablets (15 to 20 grams)
- ▶ 1 dose of glucose gel (15 grams)

Other sources of approximately 15 to 20 grams of carbohydrate:
- ▶ 1/2 to 2/3 cup of orange juice (about 4 to 5 ounces)
- ▶ 1/2 to 2/3 cup of regular soda (not sugar free)
- ▶ 2/3 to 3/4 cup of regular ginger ale (about 5 to 6 ounces)
- ▶ 1 to 1 1/2 tablespoons of honey or syrup

Treating hypoglycemia should be prompt. Always go by the blood glucose numbers, and if you are in doubt, double check the test to be sure. Symptoms are useful, but numbers are facts. Once you have treated the hypoglycemia, it is wise to check 15 minutes later to verify that the treatment resolved the issue. If not, repeat the treatment. When your blood glucose returns to normal, you may need a snack to prevent the hypoglycemia from reoccurring, and you should never begin (or continue) exercising until the hypoglycemia is resolved. Ideally, you will have an exercise partner who can offer you the proper assistance should you need it.

Glucose tablets and glucose gel are also portable, so if you are at risk for hypoglycemia, carry them with you at all times and have carbohydrate snacks on hand to avoid completely missing a meal. If you take insulin and are also taking an alpha glucosidase inhibitor (such as acarbose or miglitol), keep in mind that when you take the inhibitor, it delays the absorption of carbohydrate, so glucose tablets or gel are the best choice. If you are unsure of your symptoms or you cannot check your blood glucose level, it's better to treat your hypoglycemia than it is to wait it out.

To minimize reactions, problem solve by thinking about what caused the hypoglycemia, so you can try and avoid that situation in the future. If you tend to have hypoglycemia at certain times of day or night, discuss with your diabetes care team to determine if your medication needs adjusting.

Reducing Risks: Reaching Your Target Numbers

If your numbers are not in line with your targeted goals, your diabetes care team will recommend action to bring levels into target ranges. These actions will likely include lifestyle modifications, such as healthy eating, regular physical activity, maintaining a healthy weight, taking diabetes medication, improving sleep quality, and eliminating the use of tobacco products. The good news is that healthy eating and regular exercise can improve several of your numbers at the same time, such as your A1C, blood pressure, eye health, and lipid levels.

Part of reaching your target goals includes healthy eating and a healthier meal plan. An RD/RDN will make recommendations that include increasing fiber in your meal plan and controlling your fat intake (Week 6, Healthy Eating, page 97), which will help to improve blood cholesterol levels.

Regular physical activity or exercise can also improve blood glucose management, help control body weight, improve your sense of well-being, and reduce your risk for heart disease. People with type 2 diabetes are also encouraged to do resistance exercise (Week 5, Being Active, page 82), targeting all major muscle groups at least twice a week (preferably three times a week on alternating days). Not all activities are right for everyone with diabetes. Be careful when starting new activities, and check with your doctor if you have questions.

Besides healthy eating and physical activity, use these best practices to help improve your control, bring your numbers to target values, and decrease your risks:

To improve your A1C:
- ▶ Pay attention to the portion size and carbohydrate content of the foods you eat.
- ▶ Ask your diabetes care provider about increasing/adjusting your diabetes medication or about adding or switching to another medication.

To improve your blood pressure:
- ▶ Stop using tobacco products.
- ▶ Restrict alcohol intake.
- ▶ Reduce stress.
- ▶ If recommended, lower your overall salt intake.
- ▶ Check and record your blood pressure at home.
- ▶ Ask your diabetes care provider about adding a blood pressure medication.
- ▶ Lose weight if recommended.

To improve lipids (blood fats, such as cholesterol):
- ▶ Monitor the amount and types of fat you are eating.
- ▶ Eat more of the heart-healthy, good fats (olive oil, canola oil, fish, and nuts).
- ▶ Ask your diabetes care provider if you need a lipid-lowering medication.

To reduce risk for urinary protein (albumin, an indicator of kidney function):
- ▶ Lower blood pressure.
- ▶ Improve A1C to target.
- ▶ Ask your diabetes care provider if your blood pressure medication is kidney-protective.

To improve eye health:

- ▶ Have an eye exam (dilated, retinal) upon diagnosis.
- ▶ Have routine eye exams (dilated, retinal) every 1 to 2 years.
- ▶ Improve A1C to target.
- ▶ Lower blood pressure.

If lifestyle modifications do not help you reach your target goals, ask your health-care team about medications to help decrease your risks. Upon diagnosis, individuals with type 2 diabetes are often started on metformin if tolerated. Metformin, a medication that helps manage blood glucose and has a low risk for hypoglycemia, is the preferred initial medication for those with type 2 diabetes. In addition, you will likely require medication for blood pressure and blood cholesterol. Unmanaged numbers can lead to the development of long-term complications, so your efforts to keep these numbers in a healthy range will help keep those complications at a minimum. If you have developed complications, actively treat them with lifestyle modification, medications, and regular appointments with your diabetes care team to keep them from getting worse.

Healthy Coping: Empowerment

Empowerment is gaining the knowledge, skills, and motivation you need to succeed with your diabetes self-management. Once you have accepted that living with diabetes is going to be challenging sometimes, but not impossible, you can start learning how to set goals to make adjustments. The cornerstone of the empowerment approach of diabetes management is recognizing that you are responsible for managing your disease through choices, control, and consequences. A diabetes management plan that you and your diabetes care team develop together clearly lays out your goals for self-care. Nothing assures self-care management success more than realistic goals, a plan of action, and achievement of your goals. This will hopefully empower you to better manage your daily choices and the consequences of those choices.

An essential element in diabetes self-management is diabetes education, and part of the education process is goal setting. Diabetes self-management education is a process to help you obtain the knowledge and skill necessary to live with the disease and prevent, or at least delay, the complications. Counseling on new medications, new technology, and/or positive lifestyle changes will be addressed by your diabetes educator. Diabetes educators are usually a registered nurse, a registered dietitian, and/or a registered pharmacist, but may include other health-care professionals as well. They can assist you with achieving and maintaining desired behavioral changes necessary for optimal diabetes care and blood glucose management. Through education, you will gain the knowledge and skills necessary to problem solve, ask the important questions, and stay on top of an ever-changing therapy. Begin by asking these questions:

- ▶ What is the problem?
- ▶ How do I feel about the problem?
- ▶ What do I want to do?
- ▶ How will I do it?
- ▶ How did it work?

Using "SMART" to Develop Your Goals

After thinking about what you want to do, set realistic goals to obtain the outcomes you want for your diabetes management. A well-thought-through plan can get you the results you desire or help you learn what might work better. One method for goal setting is "**SMART**," which stands for **S**pecific, **M**easurable, **A**chievable, **R**ealistic, and **T**imebound. This example will use exercise as a goal because exercise is good for many aspects of your health and can be a doable and often inexpensive lifestyle behavior.

Specific goals focus your efforts by breaking down a lofty goal. The most common error in setting goals is that they are too general. A general goal for many is, "I will exercise more." A more specific goal with the same intent would be, "I will walk 30 minutes a day."

Measurable goals will tell you when you have met the goal. Rather than simply saying, "I will walk 30 minutes many times during the week," you can add a measurable aspect by saying, "I will walk 30 minutes a day 5 days a week."

Achievable goals are possible given your daily commitments. For example, if you work long hours and have several after-work activities Monday through Wednesday, maybe exercising 30 minutes a day, 5 days a week isn't achievable. Instead you could plan for exercising 3 days a week for 50 minutes or to only exercise in 10- to 15-minute increments on those busy days.

Realistic goals mean you have the ability to work toward the goal and make it happen. Realistic goals are unique to you. For instance, if you are having foot surgery next week, the goal of walking 30 minutes a day 5 days a week isn't realistic. You might need to set a more realistic goal, say, chair exercises.

Timebound goals have a deadline or due date. In the case of this book, two months is the timeframe you're shooting for. If you measure your progress with that deadline in mind, at the end of eight weeks, you will know how well you have done.

Use the "SMART" method as a checklist to develop your own personal goals and then record them. You may have to make several revisions before you meet all the criteria. To show that you are committed to the goals, post them in a prominent place, such as on the refrigerator or on a mirror that you check every day. Also, be sure to share them with a friend or family member as well as your diabetes team at your next visit.

WEEK 3

Making Progress —
Practice Positive Skills

As you move forward on your journey toward optimal diabetes health, you know the importance of staying on track and have the desire to do it, so keep honing your skills. Practice doesn't make perfect in this case, but it can get you as close to perfect as possible. In other words, the more often you practice positive diabetes self-management skills, the more likely they will become second nature to you. Ideally you have a strong support system or family members and friends who will praise your efforts as you take care of yourself. As you keep going, make sure you also have a strong diabetes care team to help you problem solve when adjustments need to be made.

- ▶ **Healthy Eating:** Know your nutrition facts.
- ▶ **Being Active:** Find your comfort level with activity.
- ▶ **Monitoring:** Figure out how often to monitor.
- ▶ **Taking Medication:** Learn how to maximize appointments with your diabetes care team.
- ▶ **Problem Solving:** Prepare for sick days.
- ▶ **Reducing Risks:** Learn how to prevent heart and blood vessel disease.
- ▶ **Healthy Coping:** Identify the causes of your stress.

Healthy Eating: Nutrition Facts

Eating healthy involves knowing about all of the nutrients in the food and drink you consume, not just carbohydrate. Luckily, you can get this information from food labels. Nutrition labeling of foods is required by the FDA, under the Nutrition Labeling and Education Act of 1990, which identifies the nutrients that must be listed on all food labels, other ingredients that may be listed, health claims, and standard portion sizes. The act also defines terminology commonly used on labels such as "light," "low fat," and "sodium free." The nutrition information on food labels can be found in several locations—the nutrition facts panel, the ingredient list, and other areas where health claims may be displayed. Your best source of information is the nutrition facts panel, where manufacturers provide serving size information, quantities of specific nutrients, and percent daily values (%DV). Skill at reading food labels and recognizing the nutrient content of foods can benefit your blood glucose management.

In 2016, the FDA made some changes to the nutrition facts label. The label was updated to reflect current scientific information, including the link between diet, chronic diseases, and public health, and serving

Nutrition Facts

Serving Size 2/3 cup (55g)
Servings Per Container About 8

Amount Per Serving

Calories 230   Calories from Fat 72

	% Daily Value*
Total Fat 8g	**12%**
Saturated Fat 1g	**5%**
Trans Fat 0g	
Cholesterol 0mg	**0%**
Sodium 160mg	**7%**
Total Carbohydrate 37g	**12%**
Dietary Fiber 4g	**16%**
Sugars 1g	
Protein 3g	
Vitamin A	10%
Vitamin C	8%
Calcium	20%
Iron	45%

*Percent Daily Values are based on a 2,000 calorie diet.
Your Daily Values may be higher or lower depending on
your calorie needs.

	Calories:	2,000	2,500
Total Fat	Less than	65g	80g
Sat Fat	Less than	20g	25g
Cholesterol	Less than	300mg	300mg
Sodium	Less than	2,400mg	2,400mg
Potassium		3,500mg	3,500mg
Total Carbohydrate		300g	375g
Dietary Fiber		25g	30g

Old Version

Nutrition Facts

8 servings per container

Serving size   **2/3 cup (55g)**

Amount per serving

Calories   **230**

	% Daily Value*
Total Fat 8g	**10%**
Saturated Fat 1g	**5%**
Trans Fat 0g	
Cholesterol 0mg	**0%**
Sodium 160mg	**7%**
Total Carbohydrate 37g	**13%**
Dietary Fiber 4g	**14%**
Total Sugars 12g	
Includes 10g Added Sugars	**20%**
Protein 3g	
Vitamin D 2mcg	10%
Calcium 260mg	20%
Iron 8mg	45%
Potassium 235mg	6%

*The % Daily Value (DV) tells you how much a nutrient in a
serving of food contributes to a daily diet. 2,000 calories
a day is used for general nutrition advice.

New Version

sizes were updated to reflect changes in amounts of food actually consumed. The updated label draws attention to two important elements in making healthier food choices—calories and serving sizes. You may see both the old and new versions of the label for a while as manufacturers work to update the food labels of their products.

The FDA is allowing small businesses—those having less than $10 million in annual food sales—until July 2019 to comply with the updated label. All other manufacturers will have to make the change by July 2018. Be familiar with both as you will see changes in the nutrition facts label over a period of time.

All of the information on the nutrition facts panel reflects the serving size listed. Keep in mind that serving size is not synonymous with portion size. Serving size is a measured amount of a certain food or drink. The FDA actually sets the serving sizes for all food and drink to simplify the measurement, not to suggest portion size. Portion size is up to you. It is the actual amount of food that you eat for a meal or a snack. Is the portion you eat one serving or actually two or three servings?

The calorie information tells you the number of calories in the serving size listed on the nutrition facts panel. If the serving size is doubled, then so is the calorie amount; likewise, if the serving size is cut in half, then the calorie amount is also cut in half.

The ADA recommends that people limit their saturated fat intake to less than 10% of total calories, along with a minimal intake of trans fat, on a daily basis. Saturated fat is a fat or oil from either animal or vegetable sources that is typically solid at room temperature, such as lard or vegetable shortening. Eating foods high in saturated fat is thought to contribute to higher levels of cholesterol in the blood. Trans fats may increase your risk of heart disease, so avoiding them altogether is best. Consider your dietary cholesterol intake when choosing a healthy eating pattern and limit it as much as possible. Your overall daily fat intake should be determined based on your individual need. In general, choosing foods lower in cholesterol and saturated fats is associated with reducing your risk of heart and blood vessel disease. Dietary counseling with an RD/RDN is important to help you learn more about the various types of fat, as well as your recommended total daily intake of fat. Experts recommend eating two or more servings of fish weekly (not fried), and if you have high blood lipids, include 1.6 to 3 grams of plant stanols or sterols by eating phytosterol-enriched foods. A plant-based diet rich in phytosterols is known to reduce total serum cholesterol and LDL (bad) cholesterol. Nuts, whole-grain products, vegetables, and fruits are all foods that contain natural phytosterols. There are also many phytosterol-enriched products on the market including buttery spreads that often have claims to lower cholesterol.

The ADA recommends that adults with diabetes should limit sodium intake to less than 2,300 mg (about one teaspoon of table salt) on a daily basis. In some cases, for example if you have hypertension (high blood pressure), further restriction of sodium may be recommended by your physician or RD/RDN.

Focus on total carbohydrate to determine the amount of carbohydrate in a serving. Like all other nutrition information, the amount on the label changes with the serving size. For instance, if the amount listed is 30 grams for each 1 cup serving, if you eat 1/2 cup, then the total carbohydrate is 15 grams. Once you have determined the total carbohydrate amount, consider how this amount fits within your carbohydrate goals. As for fiber, higher is generally better. The new nutrition labels will actually break out "added sugar" separately so that it is not confused with naturally occurring fruit and milk sugars. This will allow you to better evaluate the nutritional quality of foods eaten.

The amount of protein you need is based on your weight, calorie needs, stage of life, and any medical complications. Lean sources of protein, such as skinless chicken, beans with no added fat, and 90% or leaner ground beef, are ideal. Try to include fish (non-fried) that is high in omega-3 fatty acids, such as salmon, mackerel, and albacore tuna, in your meal plan at least twice a week. Other healthy choices include soybean products, walnuts, flaxseed, and canola oil. Broiling, microwaving, steaming, or grilling foods can help cut down on fat. If you do fry foods, avoid certain oils, lard, or butter. Instead use an oil high in unsaturated fats and use it sparingly.

There is no one-size-fits-all plan for the amount of protein, fat, and carbohydrate that you should eat on a daily basis. While this nutrition information can help you get started, keep in mind that visits with an RD/RDN can help you further analyze the nutrition information of the foods you are eating and help you make healthy food choices to keep your blood glucose management optimal. Your RD/RDN will work with you to develop a healthful eating plan that works for you, taking into account what you like to eat, when you like to eat, medications you take, and your goals. This is referred to as individualized Medical Nutrition Therapy

(MNT) and it means having a meal plan that includes protein, carbo-hydrate, and fat in reasonable amounts to help you maintain a healthful weight. You and your RD/RDN can also work to determine the ideal portion size for your meals and snacks. By knowing the nutrient content of food and learning how to choose appropriately, MNT is an essential part of learning to manage your blood glucose.

Being Active: Your Comfort Level

As you keep up your routine of walking your way to better health, make sure you are tolerating the exercise well. Understanding how your body is responding to exercise is an important skill to have. There are several ways to tell if you are overdoing physical activity while you are exercising. One of these ways is by doing the "talk test." Another is by using the Borg Rate of Perceived Exertion (RPE). Try out these techniques to help you evaluate your exercise intensity.

Lower-impact exercises, such as walking, swimming, or stationary biking, are often the best choice, especially if you suffer from any long-term diabetes complications that may limit your ability to be active or that can be made worse with high-impact workouts. Properly fitted athletic shoes that are comfortable and have adequate support are also essential during regular physical activity. Have good walking shoes available in the car or in your office should you get some time to walk while away from home, and make sure that you have a pair of athletic socks available. Wear clean socks and avoid those that have a tendency to make your feet sweat. The ADA recommends using shoes with cushioned midsoles (gel or air) as well as polyester or blend (cotton-polyester) socks to keep feet dry and prevent blisters from forming. You should also check your feet daily for signs of redness or trauma and get problem areas checked and treated early.

Monitoring: Monitoring Frequency

There are many options for times to check your blood glucose levels throughout the day, so you might not know how often you need to perform these checks. How often you check your blood glucose levels will

EVALUATING INTENSITY OF EXERCISE

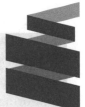

Talk Test: You should be able to talk with someone while performing an activity without gasping for breath.

Borg RPE: Rate your level of exercise effort on a scale of 6 to 7 (very, very light) to 19 to 20 (very, very hard). Try to shoot for an activity that feels in the 12 to 14 (somewhat hard) range on the scale in most cases.

```
┌─ LEAST EFFORT
├─ 6
├─ 7    Very, very light
├─ 8
├─ 9    Very light
├─ 10
├─ 11   Fairly light
├─ 12
├─ 13   Somewhat hard
├─ 14
├─ 15   Hard
├─ 16
├─ 17   Very hard
├─ 18
├─ 19   Very, very hard
├─ 20
└─ MAXIMAL EFFORT
```

Hayes C. The "I Hate to Exercise" Book for People with Diabetes. 3rd ed. Alexandria, VA: American Diabetes Association, 2013 likely depend on your treatment plan, recommendations by your diabetes care team, and your insurance coverage for monitoring supplies. If you take insulin, especially if you take several injections a day, consider monitoring your blood glucose at these times:

- ► Before meals and snacks
- ► Occasionally one to two hours after a meal
- ► At bedtime
- ► Before exercise
- ► When hypoglycemia is suspected
- ► After treating hypoglycemia (to make sure it has resolved)
- ► Before certain tasks, such as driving.

If you take other diabetes medications besides insulin, monitor your blood glucose as recommended by your diabetes care team. No matter what your treatment plan, monitor your blood glucose levels routinely to see if it is working. The key to developing the right monitoring routine is to make the most out of the test strips that you have. If you are paying for your strips out of pocket rather than through your insurance, then you may have to adjust your routine for blood glucose checks according to your budget. Work with your diabetes care team to optimize your monitoring schedule, and it is always best to rely on your blood glucose numbers as opposed to symptoms. While paying attention to your symptoms is helpful to overall blood glucose management, monitoring is the best way to make sure you are consistently staying within the desired range.

Taking Medication: Diabetes Care Team Appointments

Health-care visits can be stressful and confusing for many people, but they are important to understanding your medications, including possible side effects and interactions. Before your next appointment, there are a few ways to prepare that allow you to make the most out of your visit. To start, bring a current copy of your medication record to your appointment (Week 1, Taking Medication, page 19).

Another way to prepare is to place all of your medications in a small paper or plastic bag and take it with you to the appointment. Remember to also include any OTC medications or herbal supplements that you are taking because even taking vitamins or herbal supplements can affect your blood glucose or interfere with the prescription medications you are taking. Bringing all of your medications often helps your diabetes care team catch a number of potential causes for less than optimal blood glucose levels. Some common mistakes include taking medications more or less frequently than prescribed or taking them at the wrong time, for instance with a meal when they should be taken on an empty stomach. Another common mistake is taking a medication that has been discontinued. Bring your medications and the list of questions you have, and remember to record the answers.

Along with your normal health-care visits, schedule an annual medication review with at least one of the members of your diabetes care team. This is an excellent opportunity for you to talk honestly about any problems you are having because there are solutions to most of your challenges. Allow your health-care team to make suggestions to help you improve. Remember that you will need to take some time to prepare for your annual appointment as well, so make a note of your concerns and discuss the questions you have regarding your medications and diabetes health plan. This can help you simplify your routine, reduce costs when possible, or understand what medications you are taking and why.

Diabetes is all about self-care. Medications may be a necessary part for you to attain and maintain optimal blood glucose management, so you play the greatest role in managing your diabetes medications. The purpose of this annual review is to ask questions, so that you can improve your skills of taking your medications correctly. Possible questions to ask yourself before the appointment are:

- ▶ Is the medication schedule too complicated or too time consuming for me?
- ▶ Am I having difficulties swallowing certain oral medications, or do they upset my stomach?

- Do I know the names of my medications and understand how they all work?
- If I take a lot of medications during the day, do I often mix them up?
- What time should I take my many medications?
- Is the cost of medication a problem for me?
- If so, do I need to ask my care team if there is an alternate version of the medication that I could take or if the medication is available as a combination?

Your diabetes care team members will have the answers to your questions and solutions to medication problems you may experience. Don't be afraid to ask!

Problem Solving: Sick Days

Hyperglycemia and hypoglycemia are two problems to watch out for, but sickness also puts stress on the body. To deal with illness, your body normally produces certain hormones. When you have diabetes, these hormones can interfere with insulin's ability to lower blood glucose levels. You need to have the necessary skills to continue to maintain your levels even when you're sick. Your diabetes care team will work to provide you with sick day guidelines, so you can manage your illness at home.

If you have been given sick day guidelines, it is a good idea to review them periodically. You may want to consider reviewing them in the early fall, prior to cold and flu season. This way, you can be sure to have the necessary items ready for whenever sickness occurs.

Here is a list of suggested items to have at home:

- Clear fluids—regular soda (not sugar-free) and ginger ale
- Regular Jell-O, pudding, and applesauce
- Soups
- Crackers
- Popsicles

- ▶ Anti-diarrheal/anti-nausea medications
- ▶ Cough syrup
- ▶ Thermometer
- ▶ Pain relievers
- ▶ Cold medications
- ▶ Ketone testing strips (if recommended)
- ▶ Glucose monitor and supplies
- ▶ Notepad or electronic device to record blood glucose checks, ketone checks (if recommended), and food and fluid intake

Keeping a copy of your sick day guidelines and other necessary items in a plastic container with a lid is a great way to be certain you have everything you need in one easy-to-find place. Be sure to have a list of phone numbers for your diabetes care team and pharmacist with your guidelines, and know the best way to reach them at night, on weekends, and on holidays. Call your health-care team immediately if you have:

- ▶ vomiting
- ▶ diarrhea
- ▶ consistent blood glucose levels over 240 mg/dL
- ▶ moderate to large ketones in your urine
- ▶ had a fever for more than one day
- ▶ a fever over 101°F
- ▶ dry mouth and cracked lips (symptoms of dehydration)
- ▶ been sick for more than two days
- ▶ been unable to eat for more than one day
- ▶ symptoms such as chest pain, trouble breathing, or fruity breath

Have this information ready:

- ▶ How long have you been sick?
- ▶ What are your symptoms?
- ▶ What are your blood glucose numbers?
- ▶ If recommended, what were your ketone testing results?
- ▶ What are your temperatures?

GENERAL SICK DAY GUIDELINES

Here is an example of general guidelines for days when you are not feeling well. Your diabetes care team will provide you with specific information for sick days, including how to handle and/or adjust your diabetes medications.

- ► Check your blood glucose at least every two hours while awake.
- ► Drink plenty of fluids. If your blood glucose is high, calorie-free or carbohydrate-free beverages are best.
- ► If your temperature is over 99°, drink 8 ounces of fluid every hour while awake.
- ► Continue to take your oral diabetes medications.
- ► Continue to take your usual doses of insulin if prescribed.
- ► If you have diabetes medication prescribed to "cover" your meals, you may need to discontinue if you are not eating.
- ► It is best to check with your diabetes care team ahead of time for specific instructions on how to take your diabetes medications when you are ill.
- ► Have easy-on-the-stomach foods on hand in case you can't eat as usual. Aim for 15 grams of carbohydrate every three to four hours. Common sick day food sources that contain about 15 grams of carbohydrate include:
  - ○ 6 to 8 saltine crackers
  - ○ 1 slice of bread
  - ○ 1 cup yogurt
  - ○ 1 cup chicken noodle soup
  - ○ 1/2 cup clear regular (not diet) soda
  - ○ 2/3 cup of ginger ale

- What have you had to eat and drink over the last 24 hours?
- What is the phone number for your pharmacy?
- What medicines are you taking?
- What doses of medication have you taken (include both diabetes and other medications)?

Reducing Risks: Heart and Blood Vessel Disease

Improving your target numbers can help prevent long-term complications, including heart and blood vessel disease. You are at a higher risk if you have poorly managed blood glucose because hyperglycemia can contribute to the development of fatty deposits in your blood vessels. This results in "atherosclerosis," or hardening of the arteries, and it limits the flow of blood to the heart, brain, and limbs. Other risk factors for heart and blood vessel disease include: family history, carrying extra weight around your waist, high blood pressure, abnormal cholesterol, high LDL (bad) cholesterol, low HDL (good) cholesterol, and high triglycerides. Be aware of other heart and blood vessel diseases such as:

- Coronary artery disease: clogged arteries to the heart, which can cause heart attack or chest pain due to restricted blood flow
- Congestive heart failure: the heart loses pumping power leading to fluid buildup in feet and lungs
- Stroke: clogged blood vessels or bleeding cause death of brain cells
- Peripheral vascular disease: leg arteries become blocked, not allowing enough blood to pass, which causes pain

Prevention behaviors are behaviors and skills you can apply now to avoid heart and blood vessel disease. To reduce your risk factors, make positive changes in your lifestyle behaviors. Research shows that a few modifiable lifestyle changes can successfully reduce your risk of diabetes complications. Begin by increasing your daily physical activity. Keep your A1C below the target of 7%, check your blood glucose regularly with self-monitoring of blood glucose, and maintain a healthy body weight.

Another factor in heart and blood vessel disease is abnormal cholesterol. High LDL cholesterol and triglycerides and low HDL cholesterol are common in diabetes, so controlling your cholesterol levels can reduce your risk of a heart attack or stroke. Be sure to follow a healthy meal plan that is high in fiber and that emphasizes heart-healthy, high-quality fat and minimizes saturated fat and trans fat. Also, have your blood pressure checked at every health-care visit. For most people with diabetes, the goal for blood pressure is 140/90 mmHg or less, but the recommendation may vary depending on your individual health concerns. Keeping blood pressure within target levels will help reduce your chances of heart disease or stroke as well as decrease the risk of developing eye, kidney, or nerve diseases.

Even when LDL levels are within target ranges, the ADA recommends statin therapy for almost all people who have diabetes. You may also require several medications including angiotensin-converting enzyme (ACE) inhibitors or angiotensin receptor blockers (ARBs), thiazide diuretics (water pills), or calcium channel blockers to help control your blood pressure, and sometimes it will take a combination of medications to achieve optimal blood pressure and lipid control.

Studies have shown that aspirin may also help prevent heart disease in people with diabetes. Ask your diabetes care provider if you should take a low dose of aspirin daily. There are a number of things to consider before you begin taking aspirin because although aspirin is an OTC medication, that does not mean it comes without risks. However, a low dose of 75 to 162 mg per day may be recommended because of fewer side effects. Your diabetes care provider will consider you a candidate for aspirin therapy if you are at least 50 years old and have one additional major risk factor for heart and blood vessel disease, such as:

- ▶ Family history of premature heart and blood vessel disease (at a young age)
- ▶ Hypertension (high blood pressure)
- ▶ Use of tobacco products
- ▶ Dyslipidemia (lipid disorders)
- ▶ Albumin (a protein substance) in the urine

Healthy Coping: Stressors

Stress is the physical and emotional reaction to situations that are perceived as unmanageable, beyond your control, and a threat to your well-being. Diabetes can cause stress because it requires a level of awareness, skill, and problem solving unlike many other medical conditions. Although you may understand that changing certain lifestyle factors will greatly improve your health, replacing old habits and adopting new behaviors is never easy. Some changes you will manage without difficulty and others will take time. One step to healthy coping with diabetes is accepting that stress will always be present, but also realizing that stress is a factor for everyone.

Stress can impair your ability to do the self-care activities that are necessary to manage your diabetes, and long-term stress will take its toll on both your mental and physical health. You cannot rid yourself completely of stress, but you can learn the skills to identify and manage the symptoms. Here are some common symptoms of stress.

Physical symptoms:
- ▶ Headaches
- ▶ Muscle tension
- ▶ Back pain
- ▶ Racing heartbeat
- ▶ Shortness of breath
- ▶ Chest pain
- ▶ Indigestion
- ▶ Constipation

Emotional symptoms:
- ▶ Irritability
- ▶ Anxiety
- ▶ Nervousness
- ▶ Frustration
- ▶ Difficulty thinking clearly
- ▶ Inability to make decisions
- ▶ Sleep disturbances

There are two types of stress. First is the positive type that makes you feel energetic and more productive. You may have a lot to do, but you feel in control and exhilarated by the experience. The second type wears you out and robs you of energy. You may feel pressure from a variety of sources, including family, finances, work, and mental or physical problems. Regardless of the cause, the body's reaction to both physical and mental stress will be to increase glucose to give you the energy to mobilize yourself.

Knowing yourself is the key to healthy coping. Think about what creates or triggers your stress. There can be a number of potential causes, including diabetes treatment itself. Record the things that upset you daily, and identify the cause of your stress and how you react to or feel about the stressor. A stressor is a condition or situation that causes stress and can be acute (short-term) or chronic (long-term) in nature. Rank those things that cause you a great deal of discomfort versus those that cause little stress. The first step to alleviating stress in your life is to recognize stressors such as:

- ▶ Change in health status
- ▶ Change in job or work environment
- ▶ Change in family dynamic
- ▶ Learning a new skill
- ▶ Traffic
- ▶ Noise
- ▶ Divorce
- ▶ Elderly parents
- ▶ Children
- ▶ Holidays
- ▶ Car trouble
- ▶ Retirement
- ▶ Grief
- ▶ Loss
- ▶ Separation
- ▶ Travel
- ▶ Moving

Identifying the stressors that most directly impact you is a good start in helping you overcome the negative effects of stress. How stress affects you is unique to you, so you need to explore your individual reactions to stressful situations. Stress can be managed, but you need to recognize your physical and mental symptoms and then apply one of a number of stress-management techniques that can reduce or prevent stress (Week 4, Healthy Coping, page 76). Stress needs to be managed throughout your lifetime because of negative long-term effects on your body and emotional well-being and because stressors can also affect your diabetes health.

A certain kind of stress called "diabetes distress" is a condition that occurs when negative emotions related to diabetes care, such as checking blood glucose, taking medications, trying to squeeze in physical activity, and eating healthy can create overwhelming feelings. These unique emotional issues are directly related to the worries and burden of living with this chronic disease.

The most common causes of diabetes-related stress are:

▶ Newly diagnosed with diabetes
▶ Frustration at not reaching targeted goals
▶ Onset of long-term complications
▶ Expense of diabetes self-care
▶ Unclear goals or directions for care
▶ Poor interactions and relationships with diabetes care providers
▶ Inadequate social support

Be sure to let your diabetes care team know when your self-management efforts become overwhelming to the point that you are affected negatively. Talk with your diabetes care team about strategies to reduce negative stress. Doing so may complement your daily diabetes self-management efforts and potentially improve your diabetes management.

WEEK 4

Halfway There — What's Changed?

By now, you are probably beginning to see the benefits of the positive changes you have made, and hopefully, you feel that you're getting closer to reaching the target goals for your diabetes health. Stop and take stock. What is working well and what have you learned about yourself that will help you improve your diabetes management plan? Even if you're still not where you want to be, recognize that you can always make improvements. Take that optimism and run with it, and be sure to pat yourself on the back because you deserve it! In fact, you are about halfway through your two-month plan.

- ▶ **Healthy Eating:** Figure out your ideal portion size.
- ▶ **Being Active:** Track your exercise patterns.
- ▶ **Monitoring:** Determine your blood glucose monitoring progress.
- ▶ **Taking Medication:** Decide how you will remember to take your medications.
- ▶ **Problem Solving:** Take diabetes self-management education/training to reinforce skills.
- ▶ **Reducing Risks:** Learn how to prevent eye disease.
- ▶ **Healthy Coping:** Discover ways to reduce stress in your life.

Healthy Eating: Portion Size

These days, portion sizes are often confusing in a food service industry where smalls have become talls, mediums have become grandes, and larges are described as super supremes. It can be difficult to keep track of the nutrition facts of the foods you eat when portions sizes can change based on where you're eating. You may justify larger portions when eating out by thinking you get more for your money, but in reality, increased portion sizes mean higher calories and more carbohydrate and fat, which can affect your blood glucose management and weight. Since weight is a concern of many with type 2 diabetes, sizing up your portions makes sense. When you are working toward keeping your portions in check, the following tips may be helpful:

- ▶ Measure your foods.
- ▶ Estimate food portions.
- ▶ Package your food in single-serving sizes.
- ▶ Share a meal with yourself.

If you want to be sure of how much you are eating, use measuring tools, such as measuring cups, measuring spoons, or a food scale that measures food in grams. Start by putting your usual portion on a plate, in a bowl, or in a cup, and then measure it. Next, measure out the standard serving or the portion specific to your meal plan and compare. Once you make this comparison and note any differences, you can make the effort to scale down your portion sizes.

While measuring cups and measuring spoons are by far the most accurate, there will be times when carting around those items is not practical. In those instances, you can use your hands as measuring tools, or you can estimate your portions by using common, standard-size items, such as a tennis ball or a deck of cards. Learn to visualize these items when keeping your portions in check if measuring tools aren't an option. Examples include:

► 2 tablespoons peanut butter (ping pong ball)
► 3 ounces meat or poultry (deck of cards)
► 1 medium fruit (tennis ball)
► 1/2 cup of fresh fruit (1/2 baseball)
► 1 1/2 ounces of low-fat or fat-free cheese (4 stacked dice)

Packaging your foods in single-portion sizes may also be helpful. For example, measuring snack-type foods and putting them in snack-size bags in 15-gram (carbohydrate) portions can prevent the tendency to overeat, as well as keep portion sizes in check. Also, small zipper-type plastic bags are available that have pre-measured serving sizes on them, which may be helpful to you as well. For foods that are prepackaged, such as frozen meals, take time to review the nutrition facts label or ask your RD/RDN to help you figure out how to fit preportioned foods into your meal plan.

Scale down by requesting smaller portions when eating out, if possible. Appetizer portions can sometimes be smaller, so don't be shy about ordering from the appetizer menu. Appetizers can sometimes be rich

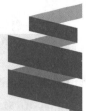

WONDERING HOW MUCH TO EAT?
DO THE "HAND JIVE"!

Hand Jive is based on a method used in Zimbabwe where teaching without any written materials is a common approach. The hand teaching method is very useful for anyone when estimating portion sizes.

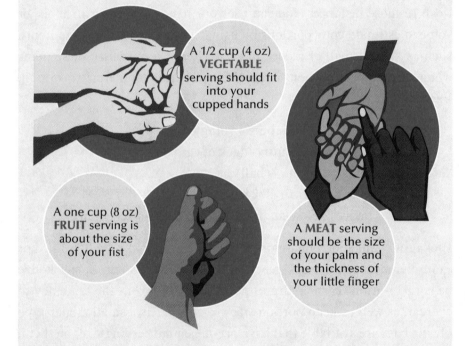

A 1/2 cup (4 oz) **VEGETABLE** serving should fit into your cupped hands

A one cup (8 oz) **FRUIT** serving is about the size of your fist

A **MEAT** serving should be the size of your palm and the thickness of your little finger

Adapted from: Wondering How Much to Eat? Do the Hand Jive! Diabetes Spectrum 1999; 12(3):177

in calories and fat, so choose carefully. Share a meal with yourself by requesting the doggy bag at the start of the meal and saving some food for later. Take excess food from the plate until you've reached the appropriate portion size and then store it to take home. Even if you don't want to take it home, it helps to remove the extra food and avoid the temptation to overeat. Taking the steps to counter ever-increasing portion sizes can help you tune up your eating habits and your health.

Being Active: Your Exercise Patterns

Your diabetes care team has probably recommended that you personally monitor your blood glucose values and keep a record to analyze your blood glucose management. It may be helpful to also record your activity levels. By doing this, you can review your progress, keep track of any challenges you face, identify any relapses in your efforts, and record how well you enjoy the physical activity.

Relating your blood glucose levels to your exercise efforts can give you information about the effect of physical activity on managing your blood glucose. Look at the days of the week when you did physical activity as compared to those days you didn't. What was different about the days? Were you busy at work when exercise seemed to falter? Was your daily pattern different? For example, were you required to sit more on days that your activity levels were lower? Focus on the days when it was more challenging for you to exercise, and then think about how you can improve. Remember that any changes you make still need to be within your comfort level. Adding even a few steps every day can go a long way toward meeting your physical activity goals. What are your ideas for things you can do to increase your physical activity? Think about things that you could already be doing on those days to add steps in many different ways:

- ▶ Got a dog? Walk it.
- ▶ Have a flight of stairs handy? Use it instead of elevators or escalators.
- ▶ Parking your car? Choose a space at the rear of the lot.

- ► Going somewhere nearby? Walk there.
- ► Kids practicing sports? Walk while you watch.
- ► Talking on the phone? Stand up or walk around during the call.
- ► Going on a shopping spree? Walk the mall as opposed to buying online.
- ► Loading groceries into the car? Walk the cart back to the store.

Monitoring: Blood Glucose Monitoring Progress

By this point, hopefully you are checking your blood glucose levels on a routine basis. Whether you are sticking to your routine or struggling to maintain it, it is important that you collaborate with your diabetes care team to monitor your progress. Questions you may want to think about on a regular basis are:

- ► How is my blood glucose management compared to my target goals?
- ► Is my overall management, based on various checks throughout the day, improving?
- ► What have I learned by checking my blood glucose levels?
- ► What improves my blood glucose levels?
- ► Are there any problem areas with my blood glucose numbers?
- ► If there are problem areas, what might be a possible solution?
- ► Can I improve blood glucose at a certain time of day without upsetting progress at other times of the day?
- ► Am I closely monitoring when my eating or exercise routine changes or if I begin feeling ill?

Once you visit your diabetes care team, *always* set a plan to follow through with reporting your blood glucose results, especially when you make changes to your treatment plan. Check with your team to see what method (drop off, fax, email, or download) is preferred for you to get your records to them. Also, discuss with your team about when you might expect feedback. Additional adjustments to your treatment plan can be made based on your blood glucose values. Don't wait; focus on timely communication with your diabetes care team to make sure any adjustments made lead to improvements.

Taking Medication: Remembering Your Medications

Have you ever wondered, "Did I take my medicine today?" Even if you are diligent in going to your appointments with your care team, remembering to take your medications daily can sometimes be a challenge. Everyone will miss a dose here or there, but many people need help remembering on a regular basis. If your memory needs a little help, there are numerous tricks, devices, and gadgets available. Once you find the tactic that works for you, you'll be more optimistic that you can take your medications on time:

1. Organize your medications in one spot.
2. Link your dose to a daily event.
3. Keep a record of when you took your medication.
4. Set a daily timer to go off when it's time for a dose.
5. Use a weekly or monthly pill box.
6. Use apps that will send reminders when it's time to take your medications.

You are more likely to remember to take your medications if they are all together and in a place you are likely to be at the time your dose is due. If you link taking your medication with a daily activity or event, you are more likely to remember. An example would be taking your medication before brushing your teeth in the morning or evening or taking them with a specific meal every day. By doing this, you will form a mental habit that makes it easier to remember.

Make a chart for yourself, and check the medication off the chart every time you take a dose. You can also use a calendar to keep track, marking the calendar when you take each medication. If remembering to take medications on time is difficult, set a timer on your watch, clock, computer, or cell phone to remind you when a dose is due. This works particularly well if some doses are scheduled at odd times of the day. Using a weekly (seven-day) pill box labeled with days of the week is also a great method because you can see the pills laid out for each day, making it easy to see if you forgot to take a medication. Monthly pill boxes are also available to organize a 30-day supply of your medications, and pharmacies sometimes will provide a service where your pills come in prepackaged doses by time of day or day of the week. If you use a smartphone regularly, you can use an app to send reminders about taking your medication.

It isn't easy in your busy and sometimes chaotic life, but taking your medications correctly is worth the effort because it maximizes your glucose management. Maintaining a consistent schedule of eating, exercise, and medications helps you to better identify patterns and adjust your treatments for optimal health. If you continue to have problems remembering to take your medications, look to simplify your medication therapy. Discuss with your health-care providers ways to potentially decrease the amount of medications you are taking. Some medications combine two different medications into one, and there are a variety of combination diabetes medications that are currently available.

Problem Solving: Diabetes Self-Management Education/Training

Your diabetes care team can help you solve problems, such as hyperglycemia, hypoglycemia, and sickness, but living and thriving with diabetes will require active self-management. Diabetes self-management education (sometimes referred to as diabetes self-management training) is important to your development of knowledge and skills to handle your diabetes on a daily basis, and you can continue this training at any point. 95% of diabetes care will be self-management, which focuses on making the right choices related to your health. The ongoing process of obtaining the knowledge, skill, and ability necessary for diabetes self-care incorporates your needs, goals, and life experiences.

There are a great number of self-care tasks that a person with diabetes must master, and realistically, simply being given all the information does not mean it will be easy to follow your diabetes care team's recommendations. Self-management education can simplify many of the recommendations by your care team and help you prioritize them based on the areas you wish to improve. A good example is the recommendation of walking 30 minutes a day five days a week. You know that it will help you lose weight, feel better about yourself, improve your blood glucose management, decrease your risk for heart and blood vessel disease, and improve your circulation, but it is hard to find the time to fit it into your schedule. While good communication with your team is vital to your success, it's up to you to consistently put what they say into practice, and self-management training can give you the skills to do that. A diabetes educator can suggest other physical activities that might be more enjoyable than walking or ways to fit the 30 minutes into your daily life. Perhaps 10 minutes 3 times daily may be doable on days you can't get 30 minutes in at one time.

Your diabetes self-management should include the skills necessary to achieve your goals and evaluate your progress periodically. A useful self-management skill is organization. Say you were given written sick day guidelines at the time of your diagnosis, but you end up not having to use them for a while. Two years later you come down with the flu or a nasty cold and actually need to use those guidelines, but you might not even remember where you put them. Training could teach you to put your guidelines and all of the food, medications, and information you'll need in one box for easy access. If you are looking to make adjustments at the halfway point of your two-month plan, try to identify your self-management problem areas, and look to further your education in those areas. Your diabetes self-management education should support informed decision making, self-care behaviors, problem solving, and active collaboration with your diabetes care team so that you have the best possible clinical outcomes, health status, and quality of life.

Both your treatment goals and your therapies will change over time and diabetes self-management training will help you make sense of those changes. This education is patient-centered, meaning it is tailored to your medical needs, your preferences, and your social environment.

To prevent short-term problems and learn to tackle them head on, see a diabetes educator on a regular basis. Ideally your diabetes educator is part of a recognized or accredited diabetes education program. You can find a diabetes educator online through the American Association of Diabetes Educators (AADE) website (diabeteseducator.org). This site will provide a number of qualified health-care professionals and their contact information. To find an accredited/recognized diabetes education program in your area, you can go to the AADE website or use the American Diabetes Association website (diabetes.org). Many insurance plans, including Medicare, pay for diabetes self-management education. Your diabetes care provider can refer you to a diabetes education program near you.

Reducing Risks: Eye Disease

Today, most people with diabetes have minor eye disorders. These eye complications include glaucoma, cataracts, and disorders of the retina. However, research has shown diabetes-related eye complications are preventable with early, regular evaluation of the eye.

Glaucoma occurs when increased pressure builds up in the eye. The pressure damages the blood vessels, decreasing blood to the optic nerve. If unchecked, the high pressure can cause loss of vision over time due to retina and nerve damage. People with diabetes are 40% more likely to develop glaucoma. Risk increases with age and the duration of your diabetes, but there are several treatments for glaucoma, including drugs to lower eye pressure.

Cataracts are opaque areas on the lens of the eye that can impair vision if they become large enough. Cataracts are more common in people with diabetes who are younger in age. If cataracts impair vision, they may be surgically removed or sometimes a new lens is implanted. Wearing sunglasses with glare-controlled lenses may help prevent cataracts, especially if you have light-colored eyes.

Diabetic retinopathy (damage to small blood vessels in the eye) is caused by exposure to high blood glucose over a period of time. There are two types of retinopathy: nonproliferative and proliferative. Nonproliferative is the most common type of retinopathy. The capillaries in the back of the eye balloon out and form pouches, but usually most people have no symptoms. Nonproliferative retinopathy usually does not require treatment, but although retinopathy does not usually cause vision loss at this stage, the changes in capillary walls may cause fluid to leak into the part of the eye where focusing occurs. This causes the macula—the area of the eye where vision is keenest—to swell, which can impair vision. Treatment should be recommended by an ophthalmologist or optometrist (ideally one who specializes in disease of the retina in patients with diabetes).

For some people, nonproliferative retinopathy progresses to proliferative retinopathy. This is more serious, and if left untreated, it may lead to blindness. With proliferative retinopathy, the blood vessels become damaged, causing them to close off. In response to the decrease in blood supply, new vessels start to grow in the retina. The new vessels are weak and can leak blood into the eye, blocking vision. New blood vessels can also cause scar tissue to grow, distorting or detaching the retina. Unfortunately, the retina can be badly damaged before you notice any changes in vision. Many people have no symptoms with proliferative retinopathy until it is too late, so be sure to have regular eye exams even if you have not noticed any problems. Early detection is important if you are experiencing eye changes. Many advances have been made in laser surgery, which has been shown to lower your risk of severe vision loss or blindness.

There are a number of interventions to avoid vision loss. Have a dilated eye exam performed by an ophthalmologist or optometrist to evaluate the retina on an ongoing basis, diagnose problems, and recommend treatment if needed. With type 2 diabetes, you should have the exam at diagnosis because due to the natural progression of diabetes, you could have been exposed to elevated blood glucose for years prior to diagnosis. After the initial exam, have a dilated eye exam every one to two years. If you have eye disease, you may need an exam more frequently, if recommended. Make positive lifestyle changes to improve blood glucose management and blood pressure control to reach your target range. Regular eye exams for early detection, improving blood glucose, and blood pressure control can dramatically decrease your risks for developing eye disease.

Healthy Coping: Stress Reduction

Identifying and understanding the causes of your stress and how it makes you feel is the first step in preventing and dealing with stress. Learn to reduce stress using relaxation techniques, biofeedback, meditation, or a stress-management program. Guided imagery and progressive relaxation are effective techniques that have been used to treat the symptoms of stress. These techniques are easy to learn through books, classes, or online research and often don't require equipment or travel. They focus on tensing and relaxing all major muscle groups in the body.

You might have used a number of methods over your lifetime to deal with stress in your life, possibly including a number of unhealthy choices. Think of ways you have handled stressful situations in the past and record these. Identify activities that seem to reduce your stress levels. Some of these will be positive and healthy ways to cope, such as exercising or spending time with friends, while others will be negative. Negative methods of coping include excessive alcohol consumption, excessive eating or sleeping, drug use, tobacco use, etc. Negative methods of coping may temporarily relieve stress, but they are not healthy in the long run. Sometimes your reaction to stress involves feelings of anger, fear, or guilt. When under stress, negative thoughts make you feel helpless and less able to manage your self-care, which can interfere with your diabetes self-management plan.

Your diabetes care team can provide suggestions on how to handle the stress related to having diabetes. You can be referred for counseling, which may help you learn to change the way you react to stress. However, because you know yourself better than anyone, it's ultimately up to you to figure out what approach works the best. Try to replace the negative with positive approaches. Don't think in terms of what you can't do; instead, be optimistic and focus on what you *can* do. Make a list of healthy ways you want to deal with stress in the future. Completing this exercise will increase your awareness of stress in your life and its causes and consequences. It will help you realize how you can successfully manage stress. Healthy ways to reduce stress include:

- ▶ Work to change the way you react to difficult situations (this will take time).
- ▶ Learn to relax, maybe using guided imagery or progressive relaxation.
- ▶ Try deep breathing exercises.
- ▶ Exercise to reduce the tension in your muscles.
- ▶ Think positive thoughts.
- ▶ Talk with a counselor or a close friend or family member.
- ▶ Keep a journal.
- ▶ Listen to soothing music.
- ▶ Learn to say no to stressful requests, if possible.
- ▶ Laugh, perhaps by watching a funny movie.
- ▶ Spend some time in nature.
- ▶ Eat wisely.
- ▶ Get enough sleep.
- ▶ Find healthy ways to enjoy yourself each day.
- ▶ Read, do puzzles, or complete a craft project.
- ▶ Embrace and maintain new positive actions (such as exercise).
- ▶ Increase and maintain the frequency of positive actions (such as self–blood glucose monitoring).
- ▶ Stop destructive actions (such as tobacco use or excessive drinking).

At your next diabetes appointment, talk to your health-care provider or another member of the team about self-care activities or other things that seem difficult and cause you stress. In the meantime, you can share your frustrations with a counselor, friend, or family member. For people with diabetes, there are potential stressors that commonly occur, including the diagnosis of diabetes, adding more medications, having to begin insulin, developing complications or anticipating complications, the risk of hypoglycemia, and taking on too many self-care behaviors at one time. When your stressors are related to self-care behaviors, be sure to share what is working or not working.

Your diabetes care team members can provide you with information about diabetes, teach you skills, help you set goals, and give ongoing support. Because there are many different solutions to problems, you should not feel as if you have failed if you are struggling. If you have tried one solution and it didn't work, your team will be able to suggest another strategy. Rarely is there only one way to deal with diabetes-related stress. People have different lifestyles; therefore, they need different solutions. It's never easy, but most tasks or skills can be simplified and can enable you to master one aspect and then add on to each accomplishment until it becomes a habit.

WEEK 5

Tackling Issues — Making Adjustments

Take the time to think about what you did well over the past month and what needs to change for the future. Your diabetes care team can help facilitate the learning process and help you take a primary role in managing your diabetes. As you make adjustments, it is important to discover behaviors and actions that you know you can do consistently or better yet, that you enjoy. You don't have to sweat heavily to increase your activity level, and you don't have to cut out all of the foods that you like in order to eat healthier. Moderation and finding healthy behaviors that fit your lifestyle are key to sticking with the changes that you've made.

- ▶ **Healthy Eating:** Analyze your healthful choices.
- ▶ **Being Active:** Schedule some resistance training.
- ▶ **Monitoring:** Look for blood glucose patterns.
- ▶ **Taking Medication:** Store and dispose of medications properly.
- ▶ **Problem Solving:** Understand preventative care behaviors.
- ▶ **Reducing Risks:** Learn about renal (diabetic kidney) disease.
- ▶ **Healthy Coping:** Determine how to recognize and deal with depression.

Healthy Eating: Make Healthful Choices

Think about the choices you've made on your healthy eating journey so far and decide how you can improve. Try to make healthy choices that you know you can do consistently. This includes tracking your carbohydrate intake, managing your weight, and figuring out the right portion size.

Balancing your carbohydrate intake throughout the day is key to blood glucose management. It is usually recommended that about half of your calories each day should come from carbohydrates. One gram of carbohydrate contains about 4 calories, so if your daily meal plan contains 1,200 calories, for example, that's about 600 calories or 150 grams of carbohydrate per day. Break that amount up based on the carbohydrate recommendations in your meal plan.

Your eating plan will impact not only your blood glucose management, but also blood pressure, body weight, and lipid goals. You can get nutrition information from food labels, but you can also find this information on various websites or smartphone apps. Because many people carry their smartphones with them throughout the day, apps can help you stay on track with your daily nutritional goals and evaluate eating patterns. Smartphone apps can provide other helpful information such

CREATE YOUR PLATE

The ADA offers an interactive tool on its website called "Create Your Plate." The tool puts an additional emphasis on an effective way to manage your blood glucose levels and lose weight (if needed). To help manage your carbohydrate intake, your plate needs more nonstarchy vegetables and smaller portions of starchy foods, and no special tools or counting required. Use these seven steps to create your plate. You can also use the USDA's Choose My Plate option as an alternative.

1. Using your dinner plate, put a line down the middle of the plate. Then on one side, cut it again so you will have three sections on your plate.
2. Fill the largest section with nonstarchy vegetables.
3. Now in one of the small sections, put grains and starchy foods.
4. In the other small section, put your protein.
5. Add a serving of fruit, a serving of dairy, or both as your meal plan allows.
6. Choose healthy fats in small amounts. For cooking, use oils. For salads, some healthy additions are nuts, seeds, avocado, and vinaigrettes.
7. To complete your meal, add a low-calorie drink like water, unsweetened tea, or coffee.

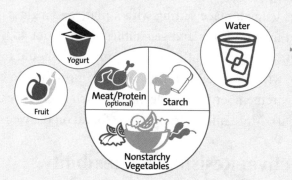

Adapted from: "Create Your Plate," American Diabetes Association, accessed November 2016, http://www.diabetes.org/food-and-fitness/food/planning-meals/create-your-plate

as calories, sodium, protein, and fat. A few useful apps include MyFitnessPal, SuperTracker, Fooducate, and CalorieKing.

If weight loss is your goal, experts recommend subtracting 500 calories from the total number of calories burned each day to lose one pound a week. Subtract 1,000 calories from the total number of calories burned each day to lose two pounds a week. You may also benefit from a visit to your RD/RDN to help you evaluate your goals and figure out where to start. Making low-fat choices and maintaining the appropriate portion sizes can also mean fewer calories and can help you meet your weight goals. For example, if you drink a serving (8 ounces) of milk three times a day, you can save 180 calories a day by simply choosing skim milk over whole milk. An 8-ounce serving of fat-free milk is approximately 90 calories, while an 8-ounce serving of whole milk is about 150 calories. That simple switch translates into 1,260 calories a week. If switching from whole to skim milk doesn't seem realistic, try 1% or even 2% milk as a lower-fat choice. Then, do the math. What other choices can you make to keep calories in check?

Managing your portions also includes the proper balance of different kinds of foods. Two examples of healthful eating plans are Choose My Plate from the United States Department of Agriculture (USDA) and the ADA's Create Your Plate (page 81). While the website (www.choosemyplate.gov) is not specific to people with diabetes, Choose My Plate reminds people to make healthful nutrition choices and to control portion sizes using a place setting with a plate and a glass. Half of your plate should include fruits and vegetables, with about 40% being vegetables and 10% fruits. The other half of your plate should include grains and protein, with about 30% grains and 20% proteins. To complete the place setting, remember to include dairy, which could be a glass of milk or some yogurt. More information can be found on the website.

Being Active: Resistance, Flexibility, and Balance Training

As you track your exercise patterns, consider adding resistance training to your routine. You can also add flexibility and balance training. As with any new type of physical activity, go to your health-care team with any questions prior to beginning, especially if you have a history of heart and blood vessel disease or eye problems. Listening to your body and safely following a resistance program is key to maximizing benefits and reducing your risk for injury. Resistance exercises include lifting weights, core stability training (i.e., pushups, sit-ups, squats, lunges, and planks), resistance bands, medicine balls, and other strength training methods. An ideal exercise program includes both aerobic activity and resistance training. Both of these types of exercise can help you preserve strength much longer. Resistance exercises can also reduce your heart and blood vessel disease risk factors, improve blood glucose management, and make your body more sensitive to insulin. Everyone loses muscle mass as they age, but you can keep more of yours by doing resistance training. More muscle equals more calories burned, even when resting, as well as a greater storage capacity for extra carbohydrates. Resistance exercises also preserve bone mineral density, keeping your bones stronger and less likely to fracture from osteoporosis.

Resistance exercises are often presented in terms of repetitions and sets. A repetition is a single completed motion, such as one pushup or one time bending and extending the arm at the elbow while holding a weight, and a set is a number of repetitions done without resting. The ADA and the American College of Sports Medicine recommend that you do resistance exercises at least twice weekly (unless not recommended by your healthcare provider), doing at least 10 to 15 repetitions per set of 5 to 10 exercises that target major muscle groups (upper body, lower body, and core).

Especially in older adults, balance and flexibility training may be recommended two to three times per week. This type of training can play an important role in fitness and function. Examples of balance and flexibility training include tai chi and yoga. Tai chi and yoga can be described as meditation in motion through gentle, flowing movements. Numerous DVDs and online sources are available for home use.

The size of a muscle is affected by the amount of activity performed. As you think about improving your strength, keep the following tips in mind:

▶ Warm up! Start by walking briskly, marching in place, or riding a stationary bicycle for about 5 to 10 minutes.

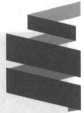

INCREASING THE AMOUNT OF WEIGHT YOU LIFT

If you have been making progress and gaining strength, you will find that you can eventually lift more weight. Muscles become stronger by lifting heavier loads. When you are able to do 12 to 15 lifts easily and comfortably, you are ready to increase the amount of weight you lift. Start by adding just one pound. Since you will now be lifting a heavier amount of weight, you will probably need to cut back on the number of lifts you do. For example, if you have been doing 12 lifts easily, you may have to cut back to six or eight lifts when you add an extra pound of weight. Gradually work back up to doing 12 to 15 lifts before you increase the weight again.

Hayes C. The "I Hate to Exercise" Book for People with Diabetes. 3rd ed. Alexandria, VA: American Diabetes Association, 2013

▶ Stretch! Go through your routine slowly without weights, stretching as you do so. This raises your core body temperature by a couple of degrees. You can also stretch in between sets of weight training.

▶ Perform sets of weight resistance training that are appropriate for you. Movement should be fluid, so lift and lower the weights in a slow, smooth manner.

▶ Breathe out when you lift weights and in when you lower weights (DO NOT hold your breath).

▶ Maintain an upright posture.

▶ Cool down by stretching for 5 to 10 minutes.

▶ Drink plenty of water (4 to 8 ounces of fluid every 15 minutes).

It may be helpful to start with the larger muscle groups (chest) and then move on to the smaller muscle groups (biceps). Try to let 48 hours pass before your next resistance training session occurs to allow your muscles to recover in between sessions. Remember that to prevent injury, avoid ramping up the intensity, amount of weight, and duration of your training program too quickly.

Monitoring: Blood Glucose Patterns

If you have been recording your blood glucose levels and checking in regularly with your diabetes care team, those are great habits to continue. An accurate record of your blood glucose helps you and your diabetes care team evaluate swings in your levels. You will want to make sure that the record allows you to see the patterns of your blood glucose numbers. If your numbers aren't meeting your goals, review the results and figure out the times of day that you need to work on as well as what affects your blood glucose, such as types of foods and physical activity.

If you do not take insulin, your health-care team might ask you to check your blood glucose more frequently for a specific period of time, such as for the next two weeks and then again the week prior to your next appointment. If you take insulin, checking your blood glucose several times daily is recommended. Keep in mind that finding blood glucose patterns is key to helping you figure out what changes are necessary to keep your blood glucose on target. It may be helpful to highlight blood glucose values based upon your target levels, such as using different colors to note episodes of hypoglycemia and hyperglycemia. Your diabetes care team may also have a format that they recommend.

Daily Blood Glucose Record

Let's say you have been checking once daily for the past week and a half. You are recording your blood glucose levels down the page on notebook paper or on your computer. Your record could look something like the one below (This is an example only and in no way reflects personal goals.):

Monday at 7 a.m.—156 mg/dL
Tuesday at 11:30 a.m.—185 mg/dL
Wednesday at 6:30 p.m.—90 mg/dL

Thursday at 7:10 a.m.—139 mg/dL
Friday at 12:30 p.m.—155 mg/dL
Saturday at 8 p.m.—85 mg/dL
Sunday at 9 a.m.—154 mg/dL
Monday at 11:30 a.m.—199 mg/dL
Tuesday at 7 a.m.—110 mg/dL
Wednesday at 7 a.m.—144 mg/dL

While it's good that you're consistently writing down your levels, it is difficult to review and figure out any patterns based on this simple list of blood glucose values. Compare the above blood glucose numbers list to the chart below that was shown in Week 2. Notice that it is easier to compare values on different days and at different times of the day in order to pinpoint trends.

	Mon	Tues	Wed	Thurs	Fri	Sat	Sun
Other Blood Glucose							
Breakfast Blood Glucose	156 mg/dL			139 mg/dL			154 mg/dL
Medicine							
Lunch Blood Glucose		185 mg/dL			155 mg/dL		
Medicine							
Dinner Blood Glucose			90 mg/dL			85 mg/dL	
Medicine							
Bedtime Blood Glucose							
Medicine							
Notes (Special events, sick days, exercise)							

In this example, you'll notice that before dinner blood glucose levels are pretty good but blood glucose levels before breakfast and lunch are high. Ideas that may help include decreasing breakfast carbohydrate intake, working with your health-care team to adjust morning and evening diabetes medications, and/or increasing physical activity.

Meter Data

Another way to review blood glucose information is by downloading data from your meter. Many meter companies have programs and software that can be purchased to provide you with a printable electronic record, and most of the programs can be customized so that they best meet your needs. This can be more helpful than just scrolling through the meter memory. Downloading your meter electronically will give automated data analysis and may include graphics to show patterns. Your health-care team should also be able to download information from your meter at each visit.

If you are relying on the meter memory at home and do not have access to an electronic record, go back one to two weeks to retrieve results and record them. Then you can make a chart that helps identify patterns. Make sure your meter clock is set correctly (both date and time) so the information you are recording reflects when the results actually occurred.

Whatever method of tracking you choose, find a routine that helps you identify patterns and also one that is doable based on your lifestyle. It may be helpful to analyze several days of data, including blood glucose levels, medications, food and beverage intake, physical activity, and other events or stressors to see the full picture. Meaningful tracking of your blood glucose numbers helps you determine cause-and-effect relationships, and then you can make the necessary changes to your care plan.

Taking Medication:
Medication Storage and Disposal

Organization and proper storage of medications is key to remembering to take them at the correct times, but it also helps your medications maintain their potency. Heat, light, and moisture can ruin your medication, so the majority of medications should be stored in a cool, dry environment. Many people store their medications in the bathroom, where conditions are often hot and steamy. These conditions cause the medication to lose potency and not work as effectively. Other areas to avoid include next to your stove, in direct sunlight, and in any place where children could see and reach them. Consider storing medications in cool, dry places, such as a drawer in your bedroom. When traveling, do not store medication in your car and remember to keep it within reach in your carry-on bags when flying.

Manufacturers of insulin and other injectable medications recommend storing them in a refrigerator prior to use. Once opened, make sure that you understand and follow the manufacturer's storage recommendations. You will find that insulin stability (in use at room temperature) varies depending upon the brand and type of insulin and whether it is stored in a vial, cartridge, pen, or insulin pump. Proper storage of other injectable medications also varies by manufacturer. Make sure that your refrigerator has stable temperatures and avoid placing these medications in spots where items may freeze.

You can also find storage suggestions by reading the labels on medication containers and pharmacy printouts when picking up your prescriptions, or you can talk to your pharmacist. The medication printout contains valuable information, including how to store each medication to maintain its potency.

Medication Disposal

As you take inventory of your medications and work with your care team to make adjustments to the medications you take, you might have to dispose of some of the medications that you no longer use. The drug enforcement agency (DEA) and local officials may sponsor "prescription drug take back days." Other options for learning about safe disposal are contacting your pharmacy or local law enforcement.

Syringes, needles, and lancets for blood glucose monitoring are considered medical equipment; they are sometimes referred to as "sharps." You will need to know how to dispose of them safely and securely to help prevent people being injured. Never throw loose sharps in the trash, don't flush them down the toilet, and keep them out of reach of children. States and counties vary with respect to regulations for disposal of medical equipment, so call your local trash or public health department to find out about available sharps disposal programs. Place needles and other sharps in a sharps disposal container immediately after use. An FDA-approved container specifically designed for the disposal of medical sharps may be purchased. These containers can be found at your local pharmacy, but other options include a heavy-duty plastic or metal container with a screw-on lid. Laundry detergent bottles or metal coffee cans may be used, as long as you make sure to properly label the container. Once the sharps container is full, never place it in a recycling bin, but follow your local guidelines for disposal. Be prepared and carry a portable sharps disposal container when traveling.

Problem Solving: Preventative Care

While complications can be preventable, some may develop rapidly and respond to treatment just as quickly. These complications may temporarily affect your ability to function normally. For example, you may have trouble focusing or thinking clearly. When you effectively self-manage your diabetes and seek regular care with your diabetes care team, problems can be avoided. Even if a problem arises, routine care will help you identify it early so it can be managed.

As a reminder, here are some things you can do to manage and prevent complications:

- ► Have a healthy meal plan.
- ► Get regular exercise.
- ► Monitor your blood glucose.
- ► Take your medications as your health-care provider recommends.
- ► Treat high blood glucose.

- Treat low blood glucose.
- Lose weight or maintain desired weight.
- Achieve blood pressure goals.
- Manage lipids.
- Take an aspirin daily, if recommended by health-care team.
- Perform daily foot exams.

Review your blood glucose records along with any other health records that you keep to see how you are doing in each of these areas. If you are having difficulties, it may be time to seek assistance from your diabetes care team. As you progress through your two-month plan, you might find that you still encounter complications. It might help to examine certain areas and see if you can make any adjustments.

If you drink alcoholic beverages, do so in moderation. It is a good idea to talk with your diabetes care team about how alcohol affects your blood glucose, especially because alcoholic beverages may not be safe in combination with some diabetes medications. If your liver is working on metabolizing alcohol, it may not be able to release glucose if your blood glucose is low, which could increase the severity of hypoglycemia. If drinking alcohol, monitor your blood glucose closely and do not drink on an empty stomach. Talk to your RD/RDN about what types of food are best to eat before you drink. Monitor your blood glucose before you go to bed, as alcohol can affect your blood glucose for several hours, and have a snack if your blood glucose is below your target range. Moderate alcohol intake is considered no more than two drinks per day for men and one drink per day for women. A "standard" drink in the United States contains roughly 14 grams of pure alcohol, which equals:

- 12 ounces of regular beer
- 5 ounces of wine
- 1.5 ounces of distilled spirits

Learn how to coordinate your mealtimes with when your medications are most active and balance the medication with the amount of food that you eat. If you are prescribed a new medication or if you are considering taking an OTC medication or herbal product, discuss how the medication works and how it will help you. Ask your diabetes care team, including your pharmacist, what effect, if any, the new medication will have on your blood glucose levels.

One risk factor for heart and blood vessel disease is an LDL cholesterol of 100 mg/dL or greater. One way to improve your lipid profile is to learn more about how it can affect your overall health and about changes that you can make to prevent complications. ADA guidelines recommend weight loss (if necessary), reducing your intake of saturated and trans fat and cholesterol, and increasing your intake of omega-3 fatty acids, viscous fiber, and phytosterols. You may also have medication prescribed if necessary to help reduce your risk.

Lifestyle changes, including meal plan, physical activity, and behavioral therapy, along with medications, are being prescribed for people who have weight loss as a goal. Achieving and maintaining at least 5% weight loss can help improve blood glucose, blood pressure, and lipids. Bariatric surgery (surgery that restricts the amount of food that goes into the stomach) may be a consideration if you have a body mass index (BMI) of 35 or greater and other conditions that limit your ability to reach your weight-loss goals.

It is also recommended to have regular dental checkups every six months. Make sure that your dentist and dental hygienist know that you have diabetes, so that they can be on the lookout for any complications. People with diabetes are at increased risk of having dental problems, such as tooth decay (cavities), early gum disease (gingivitis), and serious gum disease (periodontitis). Having good blood glucose management and taking good care of your teeth and gums helps keep your mouth healthy. Caring for your teeth includes brushing your teeth at least twice a day and flossing at least once a day.

Smoking contributes to insulin resistance, so the more cigarettes that you smoke, the higher your risk of serious complications. Smoking and diabetes is a dangerous combination, so talk with your diabetes care team about strategies to help you quit and look into smoking cessation programs in your area.

It is important to understand what preventative care is needed to help you take good care of yourself. Blood pressure checks; lab tests to check A1C, kidney function, and lipid values; regular exams; and knowing your target goals and how frequently you should get them checked will empower you to plan your care.

Reducing Risks: Diabetic Kidney Disease

Along with an increased risk of heart and eye disease, people with diabetes are also at risk for renal (kidney) disease. The kidneys remove the waste products from the blood while retaining the useful components like protein (albumin) and red blood cells. Diabetes can damage the blood vessels in the kidneys, making them less able to clean your blood correctly. Over time, high levels of blood glucose cause the kidneys to filter too much blood. The kidneys work overtime to remove waste from building up in the blood and eventually stop working properly, resulting in proteins being lost to the urine. Having small amounts of protein in the urine is called "albuminuria." This is one of the earliest signs of kidney disease and can be detected by a lab test. Your diabetes care provider will want to measure the amount of protein albumin in your urine annually. Once protein is detected, there are many treatment options, such as improving blood glucose management and blood pressure control, to prevent or slow the progression of kidney damage.

One of the earliest symptoms of kidney disease is fluid buildup (edema), often in the abdomen, chest, and around the heart. This buildup of fluid may cause fatigue, shortness of breath, or frequent urination, and many also notice their shoes and clothes feel tight. Symptoms that develop as kidney disease advances may include:

- ▶ Loss of appetite
- ▶ Feeling cold
- ▶ Poor concentration

- ▶ Nausea
- ▶ Itching

Additional symptoms, such as vomiting, bruising, weight loss, daytime sleepiness, insomnia, muscle cramps, and restless leg syndrome may occur later on. If kidney disease progresses and the kidneys lose filtering ability, you will need kidney dialysis or a kidney transplant to continue to clean waste from the blood.

If you have diabetic kidney disease, managing blood glucose and blood pressure can slow and potentially minimize the damage. Other helpful lifestyle changes include having a balanced meal plan that is low in cholesterol, limiting your intake of sodium, and avoiding tobacco and alcohol use. A low-protein diet can also decrease protein loss in your urine and increase protein levels in the blood. Work with your RD/RDN to find a meal plan that will best fit your needs, including appropriate amounts of sodium, potassium, phosphorus, and protein.

Some common medications such as ibuprofen (Advil, Motrin, and generic brands) and naproxen sodium (Aleve and generic brands) can damage the kidneys, so make sure your health-care providers are aware of your medications by taking a list of all of your medications, including OTC and herbal medications, to all appointments. Also, be aware that injected "contrast" dyes used in some x-ray procedures can lead to kidney failure a few days later, so always make sure x-ray technicians know you have diabetic kidney disease. If contrast dye is needed, your physician may prescribe fluids or other therapies to reduce your risks.

Your health-care providers will reinforce the need for medications to lower blood pressure and to prevent and slow the progression of kidney disease. An angiotensin-converting enzyme inhibitor (ACE) or angiotensin receptor blocker (ARB) may be prescribed because both types of medications lower blood pressure, can slow kidney disease, and can be helpful even in people who do not have high blood pressure. Awareness of this complication, receiving regular diabetes care, and self-management are the keys to delaying or preventing kidney disease.

Healthy Coping: Depression

Living with diabetes can be a major stressor in your life. There will be times when you are angry and resentful about your diabetes. This is common, but the kind of distress that changes the way you eat, sleep, or work may be depression. While it is not inevitable, people with diabetes have a greater risk of experiencing clinical depression according to several studies. Research suggests about 20 to 25% of people with diabetes are depressed, although diabetes-related distress is reported in up to 48% of people with diabetes and their family members. In the general population, women are more likely than men to suffer depression, and this remains true for those with diabetes. Clinical depression impacts your ability to do everyday tasks and is different from normal sadness. Diabetes-related distress and depression causes some people to act in ways that interfere with blood glucose management, such as forgetting to take their medications, smoking, making unhealthy food choices, or becoming less active.

At the cellular level, the body's response to depression is to become more insulin resistant. There is a strong link between diabetes and depression, so be aware of the symptoms so you can get the help you need. If you are depressed, there are safe and effective treatments for depression, including counseling and/or medication. Antidepressant medications are some of the most commonly prescribed medications in the country. You may start to feel better within a couple weeks, although it may take six to 12 weeks to reach full effect and for you to notice improvements in the way you feel. If you have the symptoms of depression, contact your diabetes care team or a friend or family member and and talk with them about your symptoms. Paying attention to negative emotions along with the signs and symptoms of depression are positive first steps to coping, and remember that you do not need to manage distress or depression alone.

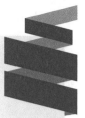

SPOTTING DEPRESSION

Have you experienced . . . ?

- ► **Loss of pleasure:** You no longer take interest in doing things you used to enjoy.
- ► **Change in sleep patterns:** You have trouble falling asleep, you wake often during the night, or you want to sleep more than usual, including during the day.
- ► **Early to rise:** You wake up earlier than usual and cannot get back to sleep.
- ► **Change in appetite:** You eat more or less than you used to, resulting in quick weight gain or weight loss.
- ► **Trouble concentrating:** You can't watch a TV program or read an article because other thoughts or feelings get in the way.
- ► **Loss of energy:** You feel tired all the time.
- ► **Nervousness:** You always feel so anxious you can't sit still.
- ► **Guilt:** You feel you "never do anything right" and worry that you are a burden to others.
- ► **Morning sadness:** You feel worse in the morning than you do the rest of the day.
- ► **Suicidal thoughts:** You feel you want to die or are thinking about ways to hurt yourself.

If you are feeling symptoms of depression, don't wait to get the help that you need. Contact a member of your care team or seek the help of a therapist, family member, or close friend.

Adapted from: "Depression," American Diabetes Association, accessed March 2016, http://www.diabetes.org/living-with-diabetes/complications/mental-health/depression.html

WEEK 6

Stay on Top — Sharpen Your Skills

Once you see the impact of improved blood glucose management on your short-term and your long-term health, ideally you will be stimulated (energized) to continue to make changes. Over the past few weeks, you've been learning and developing skills to help you better manage your diabetes. Whether it's healthy eating, taking medications correctly, or coping with emotional challenges, sharpening your self-management skills can turn short-term actions into long-term habits.

Healthy Eating: Sugar and Healthy Fats

The eating choices you make should be tailored to your likes and dislikes. A key to eating healthy is to make changes that you can live with and to be stimulated by the successes that you've already had. Because healthy

- ▶ **Healthy Eating:** Minimize added sugar and choose healthy fats.
- ▶ **Being Active:** Protect your feet as you exercise.
- ▶ **Monitoring:** Develop a plan to continue improving your numbers.
- ▶ **Taking Medication:** Evaluate the impact of diabetes medication on your finances.
- ▶ **Problem Solving:** Review your problem-solving plan with diabetes team members.
- ▶ **Reducing Risks:** Learn how to prevent nerve disease (diabetic neuropathy).
- ▶ **Healthy Coping:** Seek out a mental health professional, if necessary.

eating is a part of your treatment plan, your goal should be to learn about strategies that work best for you.

Added Sugar

When you check food nutrition information, the amount of added sugar can give you important clues on how healthy a food is. While you don't need to avoid sugar altogether, foods that contain a great deal of sugar are usually not the best nutritional choice because they don't usually contain a lot of fiber, vitamins, and minerals. In some cases, foods high in added sugar are also high in fat content. What you drink can also have a huge impact on your blood glucose, so try to choose beverages with little or no added sugars. Added sugars should be less than 10% of your total calories in order to meet your nutrient needs and stay within recommended calorie limits. The new food label (Week 3, Healthy Eating, page 48) shows the added sugars in the foods you eat.

Some sugar-free foods, such as sugar-free gum and sugar-free Jell-O, that contain less than 20 calories and 5 grams of carbohydrate are considered "free foods" because they contain minimal carbohydrate amounts. A good strategy is to spread the free foods you eat throughout the day because while they do have minimal carbohydrate, if you eat multiple servings at once, they may still impact your blood glucose. Be careful as some are sweetened by sugar alcohols that can cause stomach discomfort and diarrhea, and some individuals are impacted even by small amounts of sugar alcohols. Remember that while the content of sugar is an important fact to note, you will still want to focus on the total carbohydrate content of foods and beverages when considering your blood glucose management.

Healthy Fat

While some fat in your meal plan is necessary, consider not only the amount of fat but also the quality of the fat because some fats are healthier than others. Too much unhealthy fat can increase your risk of heart and blood vessel disease and lead to weight gain. The more that you can limit saturated fats (less than 10% of calories daily) and trans fat (limited as much as possible) and replace them with monounsaturated fatty acids (MUFA) and polyunsaturated fats, the better.

Foods rich in monounsaturated fatty acids include canola, almond, and peanut oils; olive oil; avocados; fish and nuts (almonds, cashews, pecans, and macadamias); nut butters; and olives. They may help improve your heart and blood vessel health and glucose metabolism. Polyunsaturated fats can be found in corn, safflower, sunflower, soybean, and sesame oils. They can reduce bad cholesterol levels, which can lower your risk of heart disease. Including long chain omega-3 fatty acids, a type of polyunsaturated fat found in soybean and canola oil, fatty fish (such as salmon, tuna, or mackerel), walnuts, and flaxseed, in your diet also improves your heart and blood vessel health. Remember, these foods are still high in calories, so when using in place of "solid fats"—moderation is key.

While fat-free foods generally have less calories, in some cases fat-free foods are just as high in calories as the regular version. Even if the calorie count is lower, when manufacturers remove the fat from an item, it is often replaced with sugar or a carbohydrate-based replacer, which adds to your total carbohydrate intake. Take fat-free salad dressings, for example. Hidden Valley fat-free ranch dressing is 30 calories, 0 fat grams, and 6 grams of total carbohydrate for a 2-tablespoon serving. The regular Hidden Valley ranch dressing has 140 calories per serving, 14 grams of fat (no trans fat), and 2 grams of total carbohydrate. The carbohydrate content is three times greater in the fat-free version because the soybean oil (a thickening agent that is primarily fat) is replaced with corn syrup (primarily sugar). Neither option is a wrong choice, but it is important to know how both will affect your overall meal plan.

Fiber and Phytosterols

Don't just focus on foods to avoid; think about what foods to eat more of, such as those high in fiber or phytosterols. Fiber comes from plant foods and is a form of carbohydrate that cannot be broken down during digestion. Fiber is beneficial for digestive health and bowel habits, and it makes you feel full longer. Boost the amount of fiber in your diet to the recommended amount of 25 to 30 grams daily by incorporating fiber-enriched foods. Foods high in fiber are plant-based and include fruit, vegetables, whole-grain breads and cereals, oatmeal, oat bran, beans, and peas. You may also choose to include fiber-enriched foods (such as breakfast bars and cereals) to help reach your fiber goals. Increase your fiber intake slowly by no more than 5 grams a day to avoid diarrhea, gas, and bloating, and drink plenty of water to avoid constipation.

Plant stanols and sterols, otherwise known as phytosterols, can also improve your heart and blood vessel health by reducing your LDL cholesterol because they prevent cholesterol absorption in the intestines. They can be found in plant foods, including fruits, vegetables, nuts, and seeds. The American Diabetes Association recommends 1.6 to 3 grams of phytosterols a day.

Being Active: Foot Protection

Walking is one of the easiest and least expensive steps you can take to improve your health. Is walking a stimulating and effective method of physical activity for you? Are you building up to doing more on most days of the week? If it is easier for you and your schedule, you can always break up your walks into 10-minute "mini" sessions and try to do enough sessions to reach at least 30 or more minutes a day. Building up gradually and safely is the key.

While walking has many benefits, you want to make sure your feet are tolerating your exercise and physical activity. Wear walking shoes that fit well or athletic shoes that cushion your feet and redistribute pressure, and check your feet daily for blisters, sores, itching, callus formation, or any other injuries. If you have neuropathy (damage to the nerves where feeling and sensation is altered) in your feet, your diabetes care team may recommend an alternate form of exercise for you to avoid the risk of injuring your feet, especially when you have an unhealed ulcer on the bottom of your foot, because having foot problems and amputations can greatly impact a person's activity level.

Taking the pressure off your feet, if necessary, may involve the use of some alternative forms of exercise. Alternatives include swimming, biking, rowing, chair exercises, and arm exercises. Chair and arm exercises can be found on TV, DVDs, and online. For chair exercises, use a sturdy chair, preferably one without arms. You will want the chair to be wide enough and the back tall enough to provide your body with support, and your feet should rest squarely on the floor. As with all exercise, your program should include a warmup phase before the activity and a cooldown phase at the end. Be sure to consult with your diabetes care team, or an exercise specialist, on the benefits and the risks of any exercise program and to determine the best options for your exercise regimen. Set a reachable goal for each day, and stay motivated as you continue to build up your strength.

Not only do you need to be physically active, but you also need to sit less during the day. Reducing long periods of sedentary time during your day decreases your risk of heart and blood vessel disease and also improves glucose and insulin levels in your body. Think of how much time you spend sitting at mealtimes, in the car, at work, at your computer, and watching television, just to name a few. Consider ways to breakup extended sitting times of more than 30 minutes by adding light-intensity activity like:

- ▶ Taking a walk break when refilling your water or coffee
- ▶ Standing up and moving when talking on the phone
- ▶ Standing whenever possible
- ▶ Walking around the house during commercial breaks
- ▶ Walking to a colleague's desk rather than calling that person
- ▶ Taking the stairs, if possible
- ▶ Taking a walk outside or at a shopping center

Monitoring: Fine-Tuning Blood Glucose Numbers

When you review your records and look for patterns in your blood glucose values, do you see the blood glucose levels meeting the goals that you and your diabetes care team have set? For those blood glucose levels that you are happy with, use that stimulation to continue monitoring to keep your levels within those goals. For those levels that you want to improve, think about other information that you might need to help you analyze the values on a deeper level. You might be keeping track of the date, time, and meter readings. If that isn't enough, think about other information that may provide clues, such as:

- ▶ What medications you are taking and when you are taking them
- ▶ What and how much you ate and drank (including total number of carbohydrates consumed)
- ▶ Activity levels throughout the day (time, frequency, and intensity)
- ▶ Illness, stress, or other issues, such as monthly menstrual cycle (which may impact blood glucose)

MORE FREQUENT BLOOD GLUCOSE CHECKS

There are times when you will want to check your blood glucose more often than usual. Here are some examples, but you may think of other times as well:

- ▶ During periods of stress, illness, or surgery
- ▶ If you are pregnant
- ▶ When low blood glucose is suspected
- ▶ When blood glucose levels are erratic
- ▶ When there are changes made in your treatment program, such as a change in medication doses, meal plan, or physical activity
- ▶ When taking new medications, such as steroids

As you age, it is normal for your body to change, which may require a change in your diabetes treatment plan. Staying in touch with your diabetes care team with regard to your body and blood glucose levels will help you make necessary changes in a timely manner to avoid sacrificing your diabetes management.

Adapted from: "When to Test Blood Glucose," Joslin Diabetes Center, accessed March 2016, http://www.joslin.org/info/when_to_test_blood_glucose.html

Be as detailed as possible; this information may be useful as you fine-tune your blood glucose numbers. You may want to pick a week each month to keep more detailed records to help you keep a close eye on how you are doing. If your blood glucose levels start to creep up, it might be a good idea to keep one to two weeks of detailed records to see what factors are contributing to it. Your diabetes care team may recommend that you monitor more frequently under certain situations that may alter your blood glucose management.

Taking Medication: Medication and Your Wallet

Taking inventory and proper storage of medications is more important than ever because the cost of health care is rising. Even with insurance, out-of-pocket expenses are soaring, and people who have diabetes bear a greater burden. The cost of medication for type 2 diabetes is often a barrier for people taking their medications as prescribed, so discuss any spending limits you may have with your health-care provider before he or she prescribes a specific medication. This is nothing to be ashamed of and wanting to save money on medication doesn't mean you don't care about your health. As insurance coverage has changed and medication costs have increased, many people face this same issue. Rather than just stopping a medication or changing how you take a prescribed medication in an effort to reduce costs, talk with your diabetes care team to find a more cost-effective option. There are alternatives to simply discontinuing the medications you are taking.

Begin by looking carefully at your health insurance plan and the cost of office visits, lab tests, vaccines, and co-payments. Look at the medications you are taking and compare them to what is covered in your plan, and as you review your plan, keep in mind that preferred medications are usually less expensive than others. With so many insurance plans available, health-care providers don't know what is covered under every plan when they are prescribing medications. Bring a list of medications covered by your insurance with you to the office and review them with your physician.

Your pharmacist can also make recommendations of lower-cost drugs offered by your health insurance plan. Many employers who offer sponsored insurance have an open season, a time when you are allowed to move in and out of insurance plans. If you are choosing a new plan, it is a good idea to list out and compare the prices of the services and medications you need and use at least yearly.

Shopping around for the best prices for medications and supplies can help you save money. The larger stores generally have lower prices, and some health plans offer a 90-day supply option for medications and supplies with reduced co-pays, thus reducing the cost over time. This may be available at your home pharmacy or by mail-order. When looking for lower prices on your medications, be careful about online pharmacies. There is a risk of counterfeit drugs, which can be dangerous, so look for a Verified Internet Pharmacy Practice Site (VIPPS) seal of approval. The VIPPS Seal signifies that the online pharmacy complies with state and federal requirements and standards of practice.

Financial assistance for medications may be available from some pharmaceutical companies. They offer free medication to qualified people after charging a processing fee. Ask your health-care provider or pharmacist about these programs. It may also be helpful to contact the pharmaceutical manufacturer to see if any assistance programs are available.

Another strategy to spending less could be to use combination diabetes medications. There are varieties available containing two medications in one product. Also, ask if there is a generic equivalent when a new medication is prescribed because they are lower in price. Use the time during your medication review to talk with your health-care provider about the possibility of changing costly or less effective medications.

Problem Solving: Your Problem-Solving Plan

Regular appointments with your diabetes care team will improve your ability to prevent and solve problems. At your next visit, review your target recommendations for your daily fasting blood glucose and two-hour post-meal blood glucose target levels, if applicable. Discuss what you should do when you have elevated blood glucose levels in the absence of an illness. Review your blood glucose record with your team and look for patterns in the variations from day to day and week to week. Are your blood glucose levels getting higher and higher since your last visit? Compare your target numbers to your actual numbers. It may indicate that you need a medication change or a behavior change, such as healthier eating habits, accurate carbohydrate counting, or increased physical activity.

Review your sick day guidelines with your team, especially right before cold and flu season every year. Your medication and treatments can change substantially between the time you receive your guidelines and the time you actually use them if you don't get sick often, so make sure your guidelines are always as up-to-date as possible. If you have used your sick day guidelines with success or had problems in the past, let your team know. This is a prevention measure to ensure your ability to manage a sick day at home. Be sure to get your flu shot every year to increase your chances of avoiding the flu and stay current with all of your vaccinations (Week 8, Reducing Risks, page 140).

Over time, you will develop the skills to manage possible day-to-day fluctuations in your blood glucose levels. Ask as many questions as you need to understand your diabetes plan. You have a team of health-care professionals behind you.

Reducing Risks: Nerve Disease (Diabetic Neuropathy)

When your blood glucose levels are outside of your target range, it can lead to damage to nerve cells, which is called "neuropathy." Nerves are responsible for sending messages to and from the brain telling muscles how and when to move. Nerves also communicate sensations of temperature, touch, or pain and affect the bladder, gastrointestinal tract, sex organs, heart, and every organ system. Nerve damage from diabetes is called diabetic neuropathy, and many people with diabetes have a mild to severe form of nerve damage. The development of diabetic neuropathy is often related to the duration of diabetes and can cause long-term complications.

The two common types of neuropathy are peripheral neuropathy and autonomic neuropathy. Peripheral neuropathy, or sensorimotor neuropathy, causes tingling, numbness, weakness, or pain in your feet and hands. Autonomic neuropathy affects the nerves that control your bladder, intestines, genitals, and cardiovascular system. Symptom of autonomic neuropathy include:

▶ urinary frequency
▶ bladder emptying and urinary tract infections

- erectile dysfunction
- decreased vaginal lubrication and frequency of orgasm
- early feeling of fullness when eating
- after-meal low blood glucose
- fainting
- loss of warning signs of a heart attack
- increased or decreased sweating

Many of the symptoms of neuropathy can be caused by another illness or issue, so making a diagnosis is often a challenge. Assessment during a complete physical exam includes the evaluation of sensation, temperature, position, muscle strength, and deep tendon reflexes to confirm the diagnosis.

The best way to prevent nerve damage is to keep your blood glucose as close to target range as possible, but if you are diagnosed with diabetic neuropathy, there are a number of treatments, such as medications, to decrease the symptoms. Treatment options are focused on blood glucose management, pain management, relief from depression often found with chronic pain, and protecting feet from injury. One treatment method may not be effective in everyone. Treatment for neuropathy is individualized, so you may need to try more than one method for relief. Neuropathy causes impaired sensation, leading to a loss of feeling in your feet, legs, hands, or arms, but it is most common in the legs and feet. Unless you inspect your feet on a daily basis, insensitivity to pain can often mean a cut or wound will go unnoticed, perhaps leading to infection, ulceration, and amputation. Neuropathy can also cause structural changes in your feet and toes that may require wearing special footwear and modifying the physical activities that you do.

Severe forms of diabetic neuropathy can lead to lower-extremity amputation, and hyperglycemia and neuropathic pain can predict your risk of ulcers and amputations. Amputation rates for people with diabetes are 10 times higher than for the general population. Although the risk is greater, studies have shown daily simple self-foot exams can greatly reduce amputation rates.

COULD YOU HAVE DIABETIC NEUROPATHY AND NOT KNOW IT?

If you are experiencing any of the following symptoms, talk to your diabetes care provider right away. All of these could be early signs of neuropathy:

- ▶ Tingling
  - ○ My feet tingle.
  - ○ I feel "pins and needles" in my feet.
- ▶ Pain or Increased Sensitivity
  - ○ I have burning, stabbing, or shooting pains in my feet.
  - ○ My feet are very sensitive to touch. For example, sometimes it hurts to have the bed covers touch my feet.
  - ○ Sometimes I feel like I have socks or gloves on when I don't.
  - ○ My feet hurt at night.
  - ○ My feet and hands get very cold or very hot.
- ▶ Numbness or Weakness
  - ○ My feet are numb and feel dead.
  - ○ I don't feel pain in my feet, even when I have blisters or injuries.
  - ○ I can't feel my feet when I'm walking.
  - ○ The muscles in my feet and legs are weak.
  - ○ I'm unsteady when I stand or walk, and I fall more than I used to.
  - ○ I have trouble feeling heat or cold in my feet or hands.
- ▶ Other
  - ○ It seems like the muscles and bones in my feet have changed shape.
  - ○ I have open sores (also called ulcers) on my feet and legs. These sores heal very slowly.
  - ○ I have trouble buttoning my clothing.

Adapted from: "Peripheral Neuropathy," American Diabetes Association, accessed May 2016, www.diabetes.org/living-with-diabetes/complications/neuropathy/peripheral-neuropathy.html

A comprehensive foot examination should be done at your diabetes care visit. This exam includes your diabetes care provider using a 10-gram nylon monofilament (similar to fishing line) to measure nerve sensitivity, a tuning fork to test sensitivity to vibration, palpation (touching) to check for tender areas, checking pulses, and a visual examination. Your feet should be checked at each visit, but a comprehensive foot exam should be conducted at least once a year. Taking your shoes and socks off in the exam room will help remind your health-care provider to check your feet, and be sure to point out any area of concern, such as sensitivity, pain, or a cut or sore that has not healed.

Foot care is a self-care skill you will want to develop because it's the easiest way to detect risk factors early on, preventing serious complications. If you find anything unusual or notice changes to your feet, report these to your health-care team.

- ▶ Look for sores, cuts, or cracked skin.
- ▶ Look for bumps, blisters, dry skin, corns, calluses, ingrown toenails, and toenail infections.
- ▶ Look for any swelling.
- ▶ Check for pain, tingling, numbness, or if you can't feel your feet.
- ▶ Look for reddened areas, especially red streaks, which may be a sign of infection.
- ▶ Touch your foot to feel for hot areas or temperature differences between areas (one part cold and another warm).
- ▶ Check for loss of hair on foot or leg, which may be from reduced blood flow.
- ▶ Look between the toes for redness or breaks in your skin.
- ▶ Place a mirror under your foot to clearly see the underside. If you are having trouble seeing, or difficulty bending, ask an educator to show you other ways you can examine your feet. You can also have a friend or family member help check.

Healthy meal plans, physical activity, and taking your medications will help you reach your target A1C because if you are not at your target

DAILY FOOT CARE TIPS

1. Keep your feet clean. Wash them daily with warm water and a mild bar soap. Always test the water temperature with a thermometer or your elbow prior to stepping into a bathtub.
2. Don't soak unless a diabetes care provider says it is safe to do so.
3. Dry between your toes.
4. Use lotion on the top and bottom of your feet, not between the toes. Use a moisturizing lotion that does not contain alcohol or perfume.
5. Wear the right shoes and socks. Socks should be clean, lightly padded, and fit well. Try to find socks with no seams.
6. Wear breathable materials, such as leather or canvas.
7. Shoes should fit correctly and not be so tight that they leave pressure marks. If your feet swell during the day, it may be helpful to shop for new shoes at the end of the day to make sure that they will fit well.
8. Use a moisturizer to prevent the cracking of feet. Cracks are a possible entry for bacteria.
9. Wear socks or pantyhose, not knee highs, which could cause circulation problems.
10. Always wear your shoes, even indoors.
11. Check inside your shoes and socks before putting them on. Small objects, such as tacks, stones, or other objects, will break the skin if you walk around all day.
12. Avoid wearing sandals and open-toed shoes to reduce your risk of injury.
13. File your toenails straight across and smooth the corners. Don't use scissors, knives, or razors, because you could cut yourself. Do not cut cuticles or break the skin on your feet. See a health-care provider or podiatrist for even minor treatments.
14. Avoid using a heating pad or hot water bottle on your feet.

range, you are placing yourself at risk for developing neuropathies. If you are having symptoms, report these to your health-care provider as soon as possible because early interventions can stop further problems from developing.

Healthy Coping: Mental Health Professionals

Your diabetes care team includes health-care professionals who are focused on improving your health and enhancing your understanding of diabetes. Be sure you have a current list of everyone on your diabetes care team, including contact information. Tell them if you are struggling with a recommended goal for therapy, taking your medication, or if you are dealing with stress or depression. Your diabetes care team is not going to judge. Lifestyle changes are difficult for anyone; even if you have had diabetes for a long time, you will struggle with these changes periodically. Record your experiences and take that record to your appointments to share how things have gone since your last visit. Common healthy coping problems to explore with the team are:

- ▶ Trouble understanding diabetes
- ▶ Difficulties with food and eating habits
- ▶ Competing priorities in your life
- ▶ Stress
- ▶ Family problems
- ▶ Depression
- ▶ Feelings about diabetes, such as anger, fear, or frustration
- ▶ Diabetes-related distress
- ▶ Work-related issues that interfere with diabetes self-management

There are certain coping issues that are common to a lot of people. Some problems, however, may be uncomfortable to discuss. A mental health professional can help you cope with stress, explore feelings of depression, or decrease or prevent stress that is related to your diabetes treatment and care. The best place to find a mental health professional is through your diabetes care provider or primary care physician. He or she will explore your symptoms and make the referral. Ask for several referrals because depending on your concern, you may want a therapist of a specific gender or age.

There are many types of therapists, but you will probably want to choose a therapist who has experience with diabetes, if possible. Therapists include psychiatrists, clinical psychologists, and clinical social workers. A psychiatrist can prescribe medications, so if you have symptoms of depression, your primary care physician or psychiatrist can prescribe an antidepressant along with counseling for relief of the symptoms.

Another consideration to think about is your health insurance. Many insurance plans provide coverage for mental health services, so check your insurance policy for a list of benefits and providers. Compare the providers for your plan with the list given to you by your health-care provider before you call to make your appointment. You may even wish to bring your insurance plan's list of providers to your next routine visit to ask for a recommendation proactively.

WEEK 7

Successes —
Look at the Big Picture

As you get close to reaching your two-month goal, focus on positive reinforcement by recognizing the changes you've made and take the time to congratulate yourself on a job well done. Make a list of the all of the benefits you are experiencing because of the changes you have made. Think about the health benefits, such as having more energy to participate in activities with your family and friends, but also about other meaningful benefits, such as having a more positive attitude toward living with diabetes. Continuing to partner with your diabetes care team is essential, and participation in a diabetes support group (Week 8, Healthy Coping, page 144) may also provide feedback on how well you are doing.

- ▶ **Healthy Eating:** Learn to handle the challenges of eating out.
- ▶ **Being Active:** Commit to staying active.
- ▶ **Monitoring:** Troubleshoot your blood glucose numbers.
- ▶ **Taking Medication:** Remove barriers to taking your medications.
- ▶ **Problem Solving:** Evaluate excursions in blood glucose.
- ▶ **Reducing Risks:** Develop your diabetes self-management skills.
- ▶ **Healthy Coping:** Take charge of your diabetes management.

Healthy Eating: Eating Out

It is no small task to make healthful food choices, such as minimizing sugar and eating healthy fats in moderation, meal after meal, day after day. Add a situation like eating out, whether it's at a restaurant or at someone's home, and it gets even tougher. According to the United States Healthful Food Council, the average American buys a meal or snack away from home about 6 (5.8) times each week. You will need to be creative at times to ensure you are consistently making the healthiest choices. The ADA offers these tips for eating out:

Before you arrive:

- ▶ Make reservations for your usual mealtime.
- ▶ Be prepared for a delay and bring a snack with you just in case.
- ▶ If you know your meal is going to be later than usual, eat a fruit or vegetable serving at your usual mealtime and then eat your full meal at the later hour.

To find the best place to dine, ask yourself the following questions to try to follow your usual meal plan goals:

- ▶ Does the restaurant have a variety of choices?
- ▶ Does the restaurant allow substitutions at no extra charge?

- Can two people split an entrée without an extra charge?
- Can I order dressing and sauces on the side?
- Can the food be prepared without extra butter or salt?

Start by taking a look at how often you eat out and why. Do you grab breakfast from a fast food restaurant on days that you're running late for work? Do you like to eat out with friends on the weekend? Review the places and times that you tend to eat out and decide what control you have over the preparation of food and other food choices. When you're at the restaurant, take a look at what the menu has to offer and compare the food items. Which of the options that you're considering might be the healthiest choice? Don't be shy about asking the host or server about a particular food, such as how it is prepared and what sauces and spices are included. You are the customer, so speak up; you have the right to know!

Many restaurants have nutrition information for the food choices they provide. Chain restaurants with twenty or more locations and similar retail food establishments are required to post calorie information on menus and menu boards for standard menu items. Other nutrient information, including details on fat and carbohydrate content, fiber, sugars, and proteins must be made available in writing on request. There are also free smartphone apps and free online databases available that provide nutrition information. The app CalorieKing, for example, provides this information for different types of food, food brands, and chain restaurants. Do your homework to figure out what foods are healthiest for you before you get to the restaurant. Studies show that reviewing the nutrition information and deciding what you will order before you arrive at the restaurant helps you save calories and limits the temptation to make unhealthful food choices.

Think about the recommendations that your RD/RDN has made and focus on trying to meet those goals. Items that can negatively impact your healthy eating, such as creamy sauces, gravy, salad dressings, mayonnaise, sour cream, and butter can be ordered on the side to improve your ability to control the amount that ends up on your food. Be careful and limit these types of foods, or, if you are willing, just leave them out. If your meal comes with the choice of a side, try to choose the most healthful option. To meet your goals, you can also request for meat or fish to be broiled, grilled, or baked rather than fried, and you can request that no salt be added to your food as it is prepared. To avoid unnecessary snacking, you can ask your server not to bring out the "free" appetizers, such as bread or chips. You'll be surprised at the number of places that are able to grant your requests.

Try to choose water or club soda as your beverage as much as possible when dining out. Unsweetened tea can be another healthy alternative, but avoid choosing sugar-sweetened beverages or sodas as much as possible. This will help save you not only calories and carbohydrate, but it will help prevent spikes in your blood glucose as well.

If you ate less than normal for lunch, grab a healthy midday snack that fits within your carbohydrate goals, such as an apple or a handful of nuts. If you know that you will be eating one of your meals later than your usual time, have a healthful snack at your usual mealtime. Doing these things can help you avoid binge eating later in the day as well as reduce the risk of hypoglycemia, if that is a concern for you.

Review the portion size information and stay within your limits. This will go a long way to keeping your calories in check. Many people grew up thinking they couldn't leave the table until every bit of food was eaten, so it can be difficult to stop eating when you still have food on your plate. However, it is best to always stay aware of the portion sizes when you order and to keep overdoing it to a minimum. If the portion sizes at a restaurant are larger, order from the kids' menu, share with someone else, or take the extra food home. Ask if lunch-size portions or half portions are available, and if you're at a restaurant that you know provides larger portion sizes, ask for one of the items you want to order to be brought out in a takeout container or for the takeout container to be brought out with your food. That way, you can go ahead and box up what you want to take home and not eat more than you intended.

BUFFET TABLE TIPS

► Choose the smallest plate available and focus on keeping portion sizes that meet your carbohydrate goals.

► Look for the high-fiber, low-fat options such as beans, peas, and lentils, and dark green vegetables like broccoli, cabbage, spinach, and kale. Go for the bean salads and pasta salads that are primarily fresh vegetables, and make whole-grain choices like brown rice, couscous, and whole-wheat bread and pasta.

► Watch out for dishes loaded with fat—those with mayonnaise, sour cream, and butter. Choose veggies that are light on salad dressings and heavy sauces, or bring your own healthy version of salad dressing.

► Choose lean meats, poultry, fish, or plant-based proteins and pick grilled or roasted proteins over fried versions. Make lean choices (removing the skin if present), and limit your protein portion to the size and thickness of a deck of cards.

► Choose fresh fruit and lighter options over cakes and pastries. Desserts are usually plentiful, so make the healthiest choice.

► Drink plenty of water. Iced tea with no added sugar and sugar-free soda are also reasonable choices. If you choose to drink alcohol, stay in control. Generally, moderation is considered less than or equal to one alcoholic beverage for a woman and two for a man. (Remember, one beverage is 12 ounces of beer, 5 ounces of wine, or 1.5 ounces of distilled spirits.)

► Stay in carbohydrate control. Many healthy foods also contain carbohydrates, so be sure to keep your targets in mind.

Adapted from: "NDEP Health Information A-Z," *National Institutes of Health, accessed April 2016, https://www.niddk.nih.gov/health-information/health-communication-programs/ndep/ndep-health-topics/Pages/default.aspx*

Unlimited Food

Parties, restaurants, get-togethers, and picnics often have unlimited food available for extended periods of time. Don't let the buffet wear down your healthy outlook and your blood glucose management. Instead of grabbing food as you go around the buffet table, review all of the available food choices before you make your selection. Circle the table once without a plate to see all of your options. Then you can plan what you're going to choose the second time around. Strategize to avoid overeating. Data suggest that awareness of food triggers the thought of eating. So, sit as far away from the buffet table as possible, or better yet, sit with your back to the food. This can help you make the most healthful choices possible and stick to your goals.

Being Active: Exercise Commitment

Sometimes it is easier to get motivated than it is to stay motivated to continue good behaviors. You might want to exercise more regularly and properly protect your body as you increase your physical activity, but sometimes that can be easier said than done. While there is no concrete solution to guarantee you will stay motivated to perform your physical activity efforts for the rest of your life, you are the one responsible for you!

You can start by making a commitment in writing to keep physical activity efforts going. By making a written statement that outlines your commitment, you are telling yourself that this is important. It may be helpful to make the commitment with family or friends present, those who can hold you accountable (without making you feel guilty). You might include your specific goals, the amount of activity, the duration of time you will work on the goals, and any reward system (something like new clothes or going to see a movie). Remember that you can use the "SMART" method (Week 2, Healthy Coping, page 45) when setting your goals.

Always start by setting goals that are realistic and then set more challenging goals for the future. It makes it easier to stay motivated if you are able to achieve the early goals that you set. The more you make physical activity and exercise part of your daily routine, the easier it is to stick with it. Instead of finding excuses for why you don't have time, look for ways to work physical activity into your schedule.

Seek out friends, family, neighbors, or co-workers who may be interested in joining you in your efforts because having a support system can do wonders for your accountability. Find fun sports or activities that you can enjoy together and mix up those activities when possible. If you're unable to do any weight-bearing activities or are confined to a wheelchair, think of ways you can be active by doing seated activities. Remember that sometimes you need a short break to recharge your batteries and rest your muscles. However, don't let too many days go by (preferably no more than two) because it may make it harder for you to get back into your exercise routine.

Focus on what you are doing (not what you aren't doing), and make a weekly summary of your accomplishments. You may find that recording your activity is helpful in figuring out the good things you are doing. If you find it difficult, ask an objective party, such as a friend or a member of your care team, to help you because sometimes those around us see things we don't see. When you reach a goal, think of positive ways to treat yourself. You may enjoy a massage, a new pair of tennis shoes, or membership to a health club. Rewards do not need to cost anything; they just need to help you celebrate your accomplishments. No-cost examples may include going for a hike and enjoying nature, indulging in a home movie marathon, or visiting the library to enjoy a relaxing afternoon reading. Keeping up your enthusiasm and finding ways to keep the activities fun will help you keep moving for life.

Be prepared for the unexpected. No matter how well you plan, life can change on a whim. As your routine changes, think about what you did to be successful before, such as choosing a new time to exercise, creating a schedule, or taking time to study your exercise patterns, and use these strategies to help you incorporate being active into your current schedule. Adding some extra activity into your day is ultimately worth it.

WALK FOR A CAUSE

Sometimes doing an activity for a cause can help increase your motivation. Step Out: Walk to Stop Diabetes started more than 20 years ago and is about changing the face of diabetes in the U.S., by raising funds to help prevent diabetes and find a cure. Walking a few miles brings a greater awareness to this devastating disease.

Diabetes is one of the fastest-growing diseases in the United States, and Step Out's purpose is to raise funds for research, advocacy, programs, and education. This annual fundraiser kicks off in close to 100 cities throughout the U.S., so wherever you are, gather your friends and family and walk toward a cure. Together, we can crush this epidemic.

To register for the walk or request more information, visit the American Diabetes Association website at www.diabetes.org, or call your local American Diabetes Association office at 1-888-DIABETES.

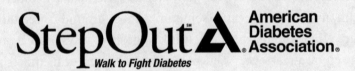

Monitoring: Troubleshooting Your Numbers

As you review your blood glucose levels to check for improvements, think about any differences you see from one day to the next. For example, if you were more active on Monday, Wednesday, and Friday versus Tuesday and Thursday, how did that affect your overall blood glucose levels? In that scenario, if Tuesday and Thursday are typically more sedentary days and your levels weren't in your target range for those days, consider what you can do to add activity on those days.

WHAT IS AFFECTING MY BLOOD GLUCOSE MANAGEMENT?

As you review your numbers and spot areas that could use improvement, think about actions that could make your blood glucose rise and fall. As a reminder, here are some common causes for changes in blood glucose levels.

What makes my blood glucose rise?

▶ A meal or snack with a larger portion size or more carbo-hydrate than usual

▶ Not being physically active

▶ Not enough diabetes medications and the wrong timing of medication

▶ Side effects of other medications, such as steroids or anti-psychotic medications

▶ Illness (your body releases hormones to fight the illness and those hormones raise glucose levels)

▶ Stress, which can produce hormones that raise blood glucose levels

▶ Short- or long-term pain, like pain from a sunburn or pain from an injury or surgery; your body releases hormones that raise glucose levels

▶ Menstrual periods, which can cause changes in hormone levels

▶ Dehydration

What makes my blood glucose drop?

▶ Missing a meal or snack, or having a meal or snack with a smaller portion size or less carbohydrate than planned

▶ Alcohol, especially on an empty stomach

▶ Too much insulin or oral diabetes medications

▶ Side effects from other medications

▶ More physical activity or exercise than usual (physical activity makes your body more sensitive to insulin and can lower blood glucose)

Adapted from: "Factors Affecting Blood Glucose," American Diabetes Association, accessed April 2016, http://www.diabetes.org/living-with-diabetes/treatment-and-care/ blood-glucose-control/factors-affecting-blood-glucose.html

It's also a good idea to do a quick total carbohydrate check on days your blood glucose levels are higher, particularly if elevated after meals. Keeping track of total carbohydrate intake is helpful to assure you are getting the right amounts for your meal plan. No matter how good you are at counting carbohydrate, food labels can be misread or portions can be miscalculated. Don't worry if that happens to you; just chalk it up to a learning experience and maybe take some time to brush up on your skill through diabetes self-management training. Check in with your diabetes care team regarding how your diabetes management is doing, what ideas you have about it, and any theories you have for making changes. Anything you do toward improving your blood glucose management makes a difference in your diabetes health.

Taking Medication: Barriers to Taking Your Medications

Everyone will miss a dose of medication once in a while due to the complexity of diabetes, and many people don't take a medication at the correct time for a number of reasons. It may be that you don't have regular work or sleep hours because of the nature of your job, or maybe you don't take or forget to take medications because you are embarrassed to take them in a public place. For many people with school-aged children, 3 p.m. begins a busy routine of homework, after-school activities, dinner, and bath and bed times. It is easy for taking your medications to get lost in the many other demands placed on top of your diabetes. Other barriers could be visual, such as not being able to read the label or see the syringe, or they could be financial, such as taking half a dose or taking a dose every other day instead of daily as prescribed because you can't afford your medication.

Your diabetes care team is under the assumption that you are taking your medication as prescribed. If you are not reaching blood glucose, lipid, or blood pressure levels within the targeted range, they will assume the medication is not working effectively and may increase your dose or change the timing of your medication to help you reach your goal. If you are not taking your medication correctly, this begins a cycle of adjustments that will not improve the way you feel or help you reach the targeted levels to prevent or delay complications. As former U.S. Surgeon General Dr. C. Everett Koop said, "Drugs don't work in people who don't take them."

Take a few moments and look at the cause of missed doses. Record your reasons and be honest when you share these with your health-care providers at your next visit. Even if you are feeling better (or worse), it is best to discuss with your health-care team before you stop taking or adjust the doses of your medications. Remember that technology, techniques (skills), and medications are continuously being improved, so there are many solutions available for any given problem that arises.

If your schedule is the issue, perhaps a change in medication or its timing can be prescribed. If remembering to take your medications is a challenge, there may be a medication that works similarly that you could take once daily rather than multiple times a day. If you have a vision or dexterity problem and can't manage without the assistance of someone else, there are a number of devices—insulin pens, magnifiers, larger print for labeling medications—that can help you. Finally, if you have financial concerns because of the cost of your diabetes medication or all your medications combined, there is often assistance for medication programs or generic brands available that can help decrease the cost.

One relatively new tool available for you are apps, which are readily available if you have access to smartphones or tablets to help remind you when you need to take your medications. Some pharmacies have created medication reminders for their patients to help with taking their medications on schedule, refill prescriptions on time, and manage pickup notifications. Three apps with basic medication reminder features and a high level of functionality include MyMedSchedule, Round Health, and MyMeds. If using apps, it is important that the name, dose, and how often you should take the medication are accurately entered. Be sure to spell the name of the medication correctly to avoid confusion.

Problem Solving: Blood Glucose Excursions

If you experience an episode of hyperglycemia or hypoglycemia, take the time after to record the steps you followed. Record your symptoms, your blood glucose level, and your actions, including those that worked and those you think could be changed or improved upon in the future. This will help you review with your care team how well you are able to handle problems at home. Recording your experiences is important to building and reinforcing skills and self-confidence in managing your diabetes.

There are many strategies that can help you keep your blood glucose within your target goals. Over time, these may be areas you will need to address:

- ▶ Check your blood glucose on a regular basis.
- ▶ Review your blood glucose records at least every two weeks to check for patterns.
- ▶ Set appropriate target goals.
- ▶ Check your medication, physical activity, and eating schedule:
  - ○ When is your medication working its hardest to lower your blood glucose?
  - ○ Do your eating times vary, and if so, how does it affect your blood glucose?
- ▶ Match medications to your schedule with the help of your diabetes care team.

Reducing Risks: Developing Self-Care Skills

When you have diabetes, there are a number of skills necessary for day-to-day care. This section will cover several key areas that cross all methods of diabetes treatment and complication prevention. By practicing and reinforcing these behaviors, you can prevent complications from arising over time:

- ▶ Learning all you can
- ▶ Self-monitoring of blood glucose

- ▶ Monitoring blood pressure
- ▶ Maintaining personal care records

Diabetes Self-Management Education and Support (DSME/S) and Medical Nutrition Therapy (MNT) are integral parts of your care. Meeting with your diabetes educator helps encourage behavior change, reinforces the maintenance of healthy diabetes-related behaviors, and addresses social, cultural, and psychological factors that could affect your health. Other factors, including physical limitations, financial status, health literacy, and emotional needs, are also addressed to strengthen your diabetes self-management skills. Your diabetes will change over time, so it is normal to periodically adjust and intensify your therapy. DSME/S can help you better adjust to changes as they occur, but it doesn't stop when your appointment is over. It must be ongoing to support your needs across the continuum.

Make your appointment for a DSME and MNT consult if you have not seen an educator or dietitian in over a year. Some of the things that you will work on in DSME classes include learning about carbohydrate counting, portion sizes, how to make healthful, well-balanced food choices, and how to safely incorporate physical activity into your daily life. Other self-care behaviors will also be covered, such as foot care and necessary screening.

Self-monitoring of blood glucose (SMBG) is another component of effective therapy. Results of SMBG allow people with diabetes to personally evaluate their response to medications, meal planning, and physical activities. Hormone levels and prolonged stress can cause variations in blood glucose levels and complicate results, so record these variations to help with evaluation and management. The accuracy of SMBG depends on the user and meter; therefore, it is important to evaluate your meter and your technique at regular intervals. Many people with diabetes are taught to use the data to make adjustments in their meal plans, exercise, or medication. Your health-care providers will evaluate your use of the data at each of your visits and will review with you your blood glucose monitoring logs for patterns in high and low readings. Those patterns are a tool to guide options for treatment decisions, so take your meter and blood glucose record to every visit.

Even mild elevations in blood pressure increase the risk of complications such as eye disease, diabetic kidney disease, and heart disease; however, research indicates that achieving your target of 140/90 mmHg or less (130/80 mmHg or less may be a goal target for some) will give you the same protective benefit as people without diabetes. One way to improve your blood pressure is to learn more about how it affects your overall health and about changes that you can make in your lifestyle to improve blood pressure control. Record your blood pressure the next time it is taken in the office. If it is elevated, you may be asked to check your blood pressure at home on a regular basis and keep a record. Devices for home use are easy to use and readily available at many pharmacies. Monitoring at home will allow you to track your improvement and the effect of various lifestyle strategies, such as weight loss, following a DASH (Dietary Approaches to Stop Hypertension)–style diet—limiting your sodium intake, increasing your potassium intake, and increasing your fruit and vegetable intake to 8 or more servings a day—or starting a physical activity program. If you are not reaching your targets, ask about medications to treat high blood pressure. Some blood pressure medications not only lower blood pressure, but help protect kidneys as well.

As previously discussed, developing and maintaining a record of your health is a valuable tool, so be sure to ask for your numbers at your visit with your health-care provider. Your record allows you to play an active role on your diabetes care team and in the important decisions regarding your health. It will allow you to see your improvements over time and identify areas that need continued focus. Patient portals, if available, are also a go-to place for supplemental information about your care, and they should continue to evolve as technology continues to improve. Your diabetes management plan is also part of your care records, providing you with the target ranges for each laboratory test and guidelines for therapy.

If you are not meeting diabetes treatment goals, ask a member of your diabetes care team what you should do to meet those goals. Sometimes, it is difficult to express your questions or you forget a question when you are in the office. To be prepared, record your questions before your appointment. Carry a notebook and a pen, a smartphone, or a tablet, so you can keep track of answers to your questions from your appointments. It can also help to bring a family member or friend to the visits, so you can be sure you heard and understood everything that is discussed.

Healthy Coping: Taking Charge

An important tool for successful and healthy coping is your diabetes self-management plan. Taking charge of the development of your plan will help you maintain positive health behaviors. It is an excellent way to make sure you are receiving the best care and allows for changes, if necessary. The plan should include your goals, give direction for your actions, and help with decision making if problems arise. It will include what you know about yourself and about diabetes, and then it will help determine and reinforce behavioral goals.

Your plan will help direct your visits with your diabetes care team. If you have had diabetes for many years, you may be satisfied with your goals. In that case, the plan will remain the same, and perhaps you can take the time to review certain aspects, such as your sick day guidelines. For the newly diagnosed, your plan may need to include self-management education since there are a number of skills that you will need to develop, such as learning to count carbohydrate or taking medications correctly. You and your team will work together to develop your individualized diabetes self-management plan, but remember that as the expert on your body, you are the most important person on that team.

Some recommendations from your diabetes care team will be easier than others to incorporate into your lifestyle. Some of the self-care tasks are more critical to your current and future mental and physical health than others, and you may need help prioritizing. Once you and your team are in agreement, you can work on goal setting. When developing the plan with your team, ask yourself the following questions:

- ▶ What aspect of self-care do I want to focus on?
- ▶ Are the goals written?
- ▶ Do I understand what I need to do to accomplish them?
- ▶ How am I going to reach my target goals?
- ▶ What steps will I take to reach my goals?

With this information, a new plan of action may be developed on what changes you want to make. You and your team will translate the goals into clear, actionable steps. Each step will move you toward your chosen goals. A successful plan will incorporate elements of diabetes self-management education and support, including assessment and planning and the evaluation of healthy coping skills and behaviors.

Take charge of your diabetes management to reduce diabetes-related stress. Actively participate in developing a care plan, learn new skills, communicate your successes with self-care with the team, and seek assistance as necessary. Your team is there to help you meet your goals for a healthy life.

WEEK 8

Moving Forward —
Two Months & Beyond

Now that you've reached the end of your two-month journey, it's time to focus on the future. Two months is a short amount of time compared to the rest of your life, and as time progresses you should expect your care plan to change, sometimes unexpectedly. When problems arise, it can feel like just as you were taking two steps forward, you end up taking a step back. Relapse in your diabetes self-management efforts is often a part of day-to-day struggles to take care of yourself, but it is important to try to stay positive when feeling overwhelmed with the journey ahead. It helps to know what causes these relapses and to understand that even if everything doesn't go exactly as planned, you should still try to do your best. It may help to connect with others who have had

- ▶ **Healthy Eating:** Look for and celebrate healthy eating improvements.
- ▶ **Being Active:** Determine if exercise has made a difference.
- ▶ **Monitoring:** Check for improved A1C levels.
- ▶ **Taking Medication:** Learn how to prepare for traveling with diabetes.
- ▶ **Problem Solving:** Review safety concerns and best practices.
- ▶ **Reducing Risks:** Consider other complications and prevention tactics.
- ▶ **Healthy Coping:** Seek out support groups for positive coping.

similar experiences and learn to develop healthy coping skills by realizing that you aren't perfect nor are you expected to be perfect.

Healthy Eating: Positive Changes

With the mindset that you are human and that you will make mistakes, take the time to recognize every positive healthy eating change that you have made, from tracking your eating habits better to making healthier decisions when eating out. You can even make a list of those positive changes to recognize your accomplishments. Are you keeping your portion sizes consistent? Are you making healthier carbohydrate choices? Are you paying attention to food nutrition information? Each small change that you make adds up, and everything you do to establish healthful eating is important. How will you know if your healthy eating changes have made a difference in your diabetes management? Ask yourself the following:

- ▶ Do I feel better?
- ▶ How do I feel about myself?

- ► Am I at a comfortable weight for me?
- ► What is my A1C?

To check for improvements, your diabetes care team can request an A1C test (Week 8, Monitoring, page 132), which gives a snapshot of blood glucose management over the previous two to three months. The ADA recommended goal for A1C for most adults is less than 7%, but your target number might be different depending on your individual needs. The closer your A1C is to your target, the better your chances are of avoiding serious diabetes complications. Healthful eating, along with physical activity and medications, can help keep your blood glucose and A1C levels in target range. Take what you have learned and put it to good use for the future. Your diabetes health outcome can only benefit from healthful eating and positive lifestyle changes.

Being Active: Evaluating Progress

Take note of the effect of increasing your physical activity. Are you making a conscious decision to add more walking or other physical movement into your day? How many steps or minutes are you up to? Have you tried resistance training? What can you do to add steps, minutes, or other kinds of physical activity as you move forward?

Several tools exist to track the number of steps you take each day. In fact, fitness trackers seem to be on many people's wrists. Before running out to buy one or getting an app on your smartphone, be sure to consider which option will best help you achieve better health. Fitness trackers may help by providing immediate feedback that motivates you to move. The right activity tracker for you will be based on your individual needs whether that's accurate step counting, calories burned, sport-specific measurements, or heart rate monitoring around the clock. Some trackers even have access to an urgent response system in case of falls or other injuries while exercising. Be mindful of precautions and claims noted by the companies that created the tracker or app, and always listen to your body.

You can ask yourself questions similar to those about the effects of healthy eating to determine if your physical activity and exercise changes have made a difference in your diabetes management:

- ▶ Do I feel better?
- ▶ How I feel about myself?
- ▶ Am I tolerating exercise and physical activity well?
- ▶ What is my A1C?

You can determine the effect of physical activity on your blood glucose management by monitoring before and after exercise (it is usually most helpful to do both to compare the difference). Keep in mind that exercise and physical activity can cause your body to be more sensitive to insulin for several hours after exercising. You need to know what activities are appropriate for you to do, the best times of day to do them, and what to do if you experience hypoglycemia or hyperglycemia while exercising.

If you get bored with a particular activity, you can always make a change. Walking isn't the only way to burn calories. Think about making your exercise activities a friend or family affair. After all, no one is too young or too old to build activity into their lives if their medical status allows. Even if you have incorporated exercise into your daily routine, it is important to break up prolonged sitting times. Get up and move at least every 30 minutes. Every little bit helps, even just walking around your chair, standing and stretching, walking during breaks, or going to the break room to refill your water bottle.

Monitoring: A1C Levels

If you have been monitoring your blood glucose levels with an accurate meter, checking for patterns, and seeing benefits, asking for an A1C is great validation that your diabetes management is improving. Since an average red blood cell lives about 120 days, the A1C is an estimated average of glucose attached to the red blood cells for that period of time. Because blood glucose levels in the preceding 30 days contribute more to

EXERCISE HELPS TO BURN UP CALORIES

If you've made progress with walking and are looking to add some other physical activities into your routine for the future, consider the following activities that are guaranteed to get you moving and burn calories:

	Approximate calories used in:	
MODERATE physical activities:	**30 min**	**60 min**
Hiking	185	370
Light gardening/yard work	165	330
Dancing	165	330
Golf (including walking and carrying clubs)	165	330
Bicycling (less than 10 mph)	145	290
Walking (3.5 mph)	140	280
Weight training (general light workout)	110	220
Stretching	90	180
VIGOROUS physical activities:	**30 min**	**60 min**
Running/jogging (5 mph)	295	590
Bicycling (more than 10 mph)	295	590
Swimming (slow freestyle laps)	255	510
Aerobics	240	480
Walking (4.5 mph)	230	460
Heavy yard work (chopping wood)	220	440
Weight lifting (vigorous effort)	220	440
Basketball (vigorous)	220	440

Determinations are for a 5 foot 10 inch male who weighs 154 pounds. Those who weigh more will use more calories; those who weigh less with use fewer calories.

Adapted from: "How Many Calories Does Physical Activity Use (Burn)?" United States Department of Agriculture, accessed October 2016, https://www.choosemyplate.gov/physical-activity-calories-burn

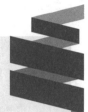

A1C TARGETS FOR HEALTHY (NON-PREGNANT) ADULTS WITH DIABETES

The lower your A1C, the better your chances are of avoiding serious diabetes complications. Check to see how A1C test results translate to an estimated average glucose (eAG) value:

A1C test result	6%	7%	8%	9%	10%	11%	12%
Average plasma glucose level	126 mg/dL	154 mg/dL	183 mg/dL	212 mg/dL	240 mg/dL	269 mg/dL	298 mg/dL

A1C targets may be modified in certain adult populations, such as women who are pregnant (typically lower) and the elderly (sometimes higher).

Adapted from: American Diabetes Association. Standards of Medical Care in Diabetes 2017. Diabetes Care 2017;40(Suppl.1):S51

the A1C than the 90 to 120 days earlier, 30 to 60 days of improved blood glucose management can contribute significantly to a drop in the A1C.

Your diabetes health-care team will determine your target A1C (usually less than 7%) depending upon your age, duration of diabetes, hypoglycemia history, and other medical conditions. For younger, healthy people with diabetes without other major medical conditions and at low risk for hypoglycemia, your A1C targets may be individualized to less than 6.5%. Depending on your age, history of severe hypoglycemia, advanced complications, multiple medical conditions, or other higher risk issues, your A1C target may be modified to less than 8%.

Your A1C level should be checked routinely by your diabetes care team. In most individuals with diabetes, it is done about every three to four months, but if your diabetes management is stable, your physician may perform the test every six months. Your A1C helps determine how well your overall blood glucose management is doing and provides you with information to help you determine your risk for the long-term complications of diabetes. The closer your A1C is to your target goal, the lower your risk for complications. For every percentage point that you reduce your A1C, you lower your risk.

Keep in mind that because the A1C detects the amount of glucose attached to normal hemoglobin, as with any test, the accuracy of your A1C can be affected by outside influences, such as medications or other disease states. However, it is a very useful tool to assist with monitoring diabetes management. Each 1% change in A1C equals the equivalent of approximately 28 to 29 mg/dL change in blood glucose. So, if you want to see how far you've come with behavior change and improvement in blood glucose management, ask your diabetes care team to measure your A1C.

Taking Medication: Traveling

When you have to take your medications correctly and at the right time, traveling takes a little extra thought, organization, and planning. You may feel overwhelmed by what could happen when traveling, but most obstacles can be planned for and resolved. Don't let having diabetes discourage you from traveling. It helps to make a list of diabetes medications, supplies, and essentials that will be needed on the trip so that you don't forget them when packing. Remember to also include items you will need to stay physically active while traveling, such as good walking shoes and comfortable socks. Always be prepared to treat hypoglycemia by packing glucose tablets or gel or a carbohydrate snack.

If you are traveling for an extended period of time or internationally, talk with your diabetes care team about meeting with them at least a month or two before your trip to develop a game plan. You may be eating at different times and eating different types of foods. Your activity level may be different from your usual routine, so try to plan ahead to include physical activity in your daily itinerary. You will probably need to check your blood glucose more frequently while you are gone to monitor closely for any blood glucose spikes. Make sure that your prescriptions will cover enough medications and supplies to last, and plan ahead so that you know what to do in case of time zone changes. Carry a copy of your medical and insurance cards when you travel, along with the contact numbers of your care team, including your pharmacy. Check to see if any immunizations are needed. If you are staying at a hotel and have any medications or supplies that need to be kept refrigerated, request a refrigerator when making your reservations.

Occasionally you may miss a meal while traveling due to missed connections, flight delays, long wait times, or arrival at a hotel too late for room service. Be prepared for all potential circumstances. Pack snacks to supplement or replace a meal that is missed. Crackers and cheese or peanut butter, granola bars, nuts, instant oatmeal, and fruit cups are easy to pack and travel well. Depending on the length of your trip and the availability to restock your supplies while traveling, try to pack up two meals per day while traveling.

Take your medications as close to your usual routine as possible, but traveling across time zones can create the potential for doses being taken too close together or too far apart. Before your trip, talk with your diabetes care team about how to handle travel day adjustments. Time zone issues to consider if you use insulin are:

- ▶ Insulin dose adjustments may not be needed if you are crossing fewer than five time zones.
- ▶ If you travel east, your day is usually shortened, which may require a reduction in insulin needs for the travel day.
- ▶ If you are westbound, your day is usually longer, which may require an increased insulin need for the travel day.
- ▶ Insulin pump users should change the time on their pump to the local time to assure the settings match the times you will be awake and asleep.

Tips for Traveling by Plane

Traveling by air? Besides the stress of tickets, connecting flights, hotel reservations, and auto rentals, you will have to deal with the Transportation

Security Administration. For some people with diabetes, this stops them from traveling by plane. Don't let it keep you from any adventure you wish to undertake.

Here are some tips that will ensure a stress-free plane trip whether it is for pleasure or work related. It is advisable to check with the Transportation Security Administration (TSA) before traveling within the U.S. The guidelines change periodically, so make sure you have the most up-to-date versions. If you are traveling internationally, it is a good idea to check with the companies that you have booked.

▶ Be sure to wear a medical ID bracelet or necklace identifying that you have diabetes in case of an emergency.

▶ Obtain copies of all your prescriptions, packing them in your carry-on bag in case you need a refill while away from home.

▶ The name and phone number of your pharmacy and diabetes care team should also be included somewhere that you have access to at all times.

▶ Carry your medications in your carry-on bag to prevent loss in your checked luggage or separation in the case of a mislaid bag.

▶ Be sure to take the prescription label for your diabetes supplies (for example, the pharmacy label is found on the box of injectable medications).

▶ It is a good idea to ask for a letter from your doctor that includes your name, your diagnosis of diabetes, and a list of all your medications and supplies. Supplies may include medication, injectable devices (syringes, needles, pens, etc.), blood glucose monitoring supplies (strips, lancets, etc.), insulin pump supplies (infusion sets, reservoirs, insulin, etc.), or continuous glucose sensor supplies. Have your physician sign and date the letter.

▶ If you wear an insulin pump, many of the insulin pump companies (for a small fee) will provide you with a loaner pump when traveling on a cruise, to Hawaii, Alaska, or an international location.

- Insulin pump users should have a backup plan for potential pump malfunction, such as having insulin syringes available or a prescription for long-acting (basal) insulin.
- Keep plenty of healthy snacks and treatment for hypoglycemia with you. Flights may be delayed, causing you to miss a meal.
- Carrying a refillable water bottle with you when traveling will save on expenses and decrease the temptation to purchase sugar-sweetened beverages.

It is important to keep your medical items in your carry-on luggage. Separate out medications, supplies, and equipment related to your diabetes and tell the TSA agent at the security gate about your needs. Separate your medications from your other packed items before the screening process. Learning the guidelines for air travel before you go can help relieve any apprehensions you may have about traveling.

Problem Solving: Best Practices for Safety

Having diabetes can put you at risk, so as a safety precaution, it is important to wear some type of diabetes identification to alert others that you have diabetes in the event that you cannot speak for yourself. Your identification should have a medical emblem that will clearly stand out. Diabetes identification comes in a wide variety, giving you many choices. Medical jewelry is available in bracelets, necklaces, and pendants for both men and women, and the jewelry can be found in sterling silver, 10 or 14 karat gold, nylon, or leather. If you have a more active lifestyle, you may want a durable sport band identification made of nylon or leather cuffs with an identification faceplate. Medical identification is also readily available at a wide range of prices. These can be found in a number of diabetes magazines and journals, various websites, at your pharmacy, at department store jewelry counters, or on order forms in your health-care providers' offices.

Even when wearing diabetes identification, it is important to educate those around you on how to recognize your usual symptoms and how

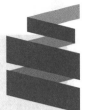

TSA-PERMITTED LIQUIDS FOR PERSONS WITH MEDICAL CONDITIONS

The TSA permits prescription liquid medications and other liquids needed by people with medical conditions that include:

▶ All prescription and OTC medications (liquids, creams, gels, and aerosols) for medical purposes

▶ Liquids including water, juice, or liquid nutrition or gels for a medical condition

▶ Ice packs or freezer packs needed to cool medical-related items for medical conditions must be completely solid at the security checkpoint

▶ Gels or frozen liquids needed to cool medical-related items for medical conditions

If the liquid medications are in volumes larger than 3.4 ounces or 100 milliliters, they must be screened separately and may not be placed in a quart-size bag, and they must be declared to the TSA officer. A declaration can be made verbally, in writing, or by a person's traveling companion. Declared liquids must be kept separate from all other property and submitted for x-ray screening. If you inform the TSA officer that you do not want items x-rayed, additional screening procedures will be undertaken to ensure safety.

Adapted from: "Disabilities and Medical Conditions," Transportation Security Administration, accessed April 2016, www.tsa.gov/travelers/airtravel/specialneeds/index.shtm

to respond in case of a severe low blood glucose level. Be sure that your family, friends, coworkers, and other people that you trust know how to recognize and treat your hypoglycemia. Don't be shy. They will be happy to help. It may even be helpful to carry a short list of instructions with you in case of an emergency.

When you have diabetes, driving is a safety concern you need to consider. Be aware that many states require identification of diabetes on the license. If you take medication to lower your blood glucose, some special precautions should be addressed. No one treated with oral agents or insulin should travel without readily available snacks or quick-acting carbohydrates, so be prepared and keep snacks in the car. As a precaution, the best practice is always carrying a pure form of glucose with you, such as glucose tablets or gel, in case of low blood glucose reactions. They can be found in your pharmacy and come in a large variety of flavors and sizes. Glucose tablets are preferred when storing supplies in your car during hot or humid weather. Check your blood glucose level prior to driving, and when you are traveling long distances by car, stop and check your blood glucose at regular intervals. Do not skip or delay meals while driving. If you start experiencing symptoms, pull the car off the road, check your blood glucose, treat, and recheck before driving. Having a cell phone available in case of emergencies is a good safety measure. An accident caused by hypoglycemia is still the responsibility of the driver, so take action quickly if you feel symptomatic while driving. Take these same precautions when driving boats, motorcycles, three wheelers, snowmobiles, and other powered vehicles.

Reducing Risks: Other Complications and Prevention Tactics

If not managed properly, diabetes can lead to serious long-term complications. While keeping your levels at your target goals and checking in regularly with your care team helps significantly with prevention, there are other ways to protect your health and prevent risks.

Immunization and Vaccinations

It is important to protect your health from certain illnesses by keeping your vaccinations up-to-date. For extra protection, encourage the people that you live with or spend most of your time with to do the same. Diabetes, even if well managed, can make it harder for your immune system to fight infections. Adults can get vaccines at their doctors' offices, pharmacies, workplaces, health departments, and other locations, so talk with your diabetes care team if you have any history of allergic reactions to any of the vaccines.

The following vaccinations are recommended:

► **Hepatitis B vaccine:** People with diabetes have a higher risk of getting Hepatitis B (HepB), which can cause cirrhosis (scaring of the liver), liver failure, and liver cancer. The Hepatitis B vaccine is administered in a series of three and protects against HepB infection. It is recommended for all adults with diabetes.

► **Influenza vaccine:** People with diabetes are also at risk for serious complications from the flu. Influenza is a serious disease that accounts for hospitalizations and deaths each year. Getting the flu vaccine may make your illness less severe and reduce your risk of hospitalization if you do get sick. The virus changes every year, which is one reason why vaccination against influenza is recommended annually at the beginning of the flu season. When all adults with diabetes get vaccinated, it protects them and helps prevent the flu from spreading. There are different types of influenza vaccines. Injectable flu vaccine is preferred as the nasal spray flu mist is currently not recommended for use in people with diabetes due to safety concerns. Talk with your health-care team about which one is right for you.

► **Pneumovax and Prevnar vaccines:** To protect yourself from bacterial infections such as pneumonia, as well as ear infections, meningitis, and bloodstream infections, the Pneumococcal polysaccharide 23 (Pneumovax) and Pneumococcal conjugate 13 (Prevnar 13) vaccines are recommended. If you are 65 years of age or older, you will need a dose of Prevnar, unless you have already received a dose of Pneumovax within the last year because Prevnar and Pneumovax are usually spaced one year apart. You may only need one dose of each. Your diabetes care team may also recommend vaccination before the age of 65 for specific populations.

- ▶ **Tdap vaccine:** Tdap vaccines can protect you from the diseases of tetanus, diphtheria, and pertussis. One dose is routinely given at age 11 or 12. If you did not get Tdap at that age, talk with your diabetes care team about your needs. Another booster called Td (tetanus and diphtheria) should be given every ten years.
- ▶ **Zoster vaccine:** The Zoster vaccine reduces your risk of developing shingles, and it is recommended for people aged 60 years and older. Even people who have had shingles can receive the vaccine to protect against future infection.

Vaccine side effects are usually mild and go away on their own, and severe side effects are rare. Discuss any concerns that you may have with your diabetes care team.

Prepregnancy Counseling

Women with diabetes considering pregnancy need to be seen by a interdisciplinary team, including a diabetes care provider, obstetrician, pediatrician or neonatologist, RD/RDN, and diabetes educator, for evaluation. Those meeting with a interdisciplinary team will be evaluated and treated for long-term complications of diabetes. The team will review all medications currently taken as part of preconception care, and it will also advise that your A1C should be as close to normal as possible before conception. Because of this recommendation, if you are a woman with diabetes of childbearing age, you should be informed regarding the need for good blood glucose management, and contraception is suggested until normal sustained blood glucose is achieved. Good blood pressure control is also advised. Statins and some blood pressure medications are not safe for use during pregnancy and should be adjusted prior to conceiving. Some might consider a preconception program that includes diabetes self-management education, intensified insulin therapy (as needed), and self-monitoring blood glucose in preparation for pregnancy.

Sexual Dysfunction

Diabetes can impact both women and men's sex lives. If you find that you no longer enjoy sex or have problems being able to engage in sexual intercourse, it is normal to feel upset. Don't be embarrassed. Talk openly with your partner and find someone on your diabetes care team that you are comfortable talking with. Ask questions about medications available or counseling that may help.

Some women with diabetes may find that changes in blood glucose levels may cause them to feel more tired and irritable, leading to less desire for sex. Women with neuropathy may experience issues with vaginal dryness leading to painful intercourse, low libido, and difficulty reaching orgasms, or these changes may occur with normal aging and menopause. This may cause feelings of anger or depression, but don't give up! It is important to know that sexual problems do not occur in everyone and that diabetes lifestyle changes along with counseling, medication, and other treatment options are available.

Sexual dysfunction is also a frequent occurrence in men with diabetes. In fact, they are twice as likely to develop erectile dysfunction (ED). ED is caused by damage to the blood vessels and nerves over many years and presents with a lack of a firm and sustained erection for intercourse. In general, libido and ejaculatory function are not affected. There may be several reasons for the development of ED. Diabetes can damage the nerves in the penis, preventing an erection even if you are interested in sexual activity. Diabetes can also damage the blood vessels in the penis, not allowing blood to reach the area during sexual arousal, shortening the duration of the erection. Other factors can be side effects of some medications, such as high blood pressure medications, beta-blockers, or antidepressants. Ask your health-care team if ED is a side effect of any of your medications as they may be able to make adjustments in your medications without compromising therapy. Alcohol, smoking, being overweight, being inactive, stress, and illness can also increase the risk of ED, along with conditions like prostate problems or complications from bladder surgery. Talk with your health-care team if you are experiencing difficulties. ED may be difficult or embarrassing to talk about, but your diabetes care team is made up of professionals who are there to help you.

There are a variety of treatments for ED including medications (Cialis, Levitra, and Viagra), prostaglandin suppositories that are inserted into the tip of the penis, injections that are taken before sexual activity, and implants or surgery to repair blood vessels to increase blood flow to the penis. Remember that if you have a prescription or take nitroglycerin, it is not safe to take with some of the medications prescribed for ED. Other diabetes lifestyle changes you are incorporating may also help. Couple counseling, relaxation techniques, and stress reduction techniques may decrease your anxiety about your symptoms.

Healthy Coping: Support Groups

Sometimes it can feel like family or friends who do not have diabetes cannot understand how you are feeling. If you have recently been diagnosed, you may feel overwhelmed with everything you have to learn and incorporate into your daily life. If you have had diabetes for several years, you may be concerned because you have started to develop some complications. You might be dealing with stress or depression, and you might not feel empowered to make the right choices. For many with diabetes, meeting, talking, and connecting with others who have the disease can be a liberating experience. Knowing that other people deal with similar challenges will validate your thoughts, so if you need to connect with others with diabetes, a support group may be the answer.

There are a number of support groups available in most communities. Support groups maintain personal contact and can provide information and a wealth of experiences. Support groups are open to free expression without criticism or interruptions, and they are a safe environment to express how you are feeling and provide encouragement to others. Relating to others with similar issues can help empower you to take care of yourself and learn positive ways to deal with issues that come up. While face-to-face support groups are the most common, other

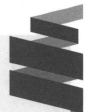

SUPPORT AT YOUR FINGERTIPS

These online diabetes communities offer chats, blogs, live Q&A sessions, and more.

- ► ADA's diabetes.org message boards
- ► DiabetesDaily.com
- ► TuDiabetes.org

Adapted from: Neithercott T. "Peer Support Helps with Diabetes Control." Diabetes Forecast, *August 2014*

support groups may include phone support (talking and/or texting) or online support (websites with specific forums). Social media is also a form of online support that has become very popular, including Facebook and Twitter. Always be cautious with sharing personal information, however. Any medical advice you receive should be verified with one of the members of your health-care team.

Your diabetes educator or diabetes care team member can tell you about support groups in your area. You can also find local support groups by checking your local papers for announcements of meetings, or calling your local hospital. You can also call your local American Diabetes Association affiliate to find support groups in your area, and if you live in an area without regular support groups or you are homebound, you can still connect with others via the ADA website, www.diabetes.org.

CONCLUSION

Look How Far You've Come!

Step back and look how far you have come with your efforts to improve your lifestyle to enhance your diabetes management. It is important to pat yourself on the back for whatever changes in behavior you have accomplished. Always give yourself the credit you deserve. There is so much you need to know and do to take care of yourself. Not only do you need to understand the information, but you have to be able translate the information into habits that become part of your daily routine. Think of all of the effort that you have put into learning what you need to know and what you need to do to take care of yourself. Sometimes it can be overwhelming, but in the end it is worth it.

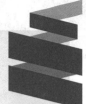

PARTING WORDS TO REMEMBER ABOUT YOUR SELF-CARE PLAN

- ▶ It does not promise beauty, but it will improve your health.
- ▶ It is not a quick process, but slow and methodical.
- ▶ It is not easy, but often difficult and sometimes painful.
- ▶ It does not tell you what to do, but helps you decide what is worth doing.
- ▶ It does not take responsibility for your choices, but offers information and support so you can make informed choices.
- ▶ It is not prepackaged, but a custom-designed program for you by you.
- ▶ It does not rely on external forces, but seeks to help you discover the forces within yourself.
- ▶ It does not judge your circumstances, but helps you live with them.
- ▶ It does not fix your problems, but offers tools to solve them.
- ▶ It does not simplify, but acknowledges the complexity.
- ▶ It is not an easy sell, but a path to real and lasting change.

Adapted from: Adolfsson B, Arnold, MS. Behavioral Approaches to Treating Obesity. 2nd ed. Alexandria, VA: American Diabetes Association, 2011

Reward yourself! Try and establish a reward system that does not prevent you from focusing on your goal. For example, going to an all-you-can-eat buffet may not be the right reward to keep you on track; however, rewarding yourself with a membership to a gym or getting a massage might be just what the doctor ordered.

Keep in mind that your lifestyle changes require day-to-day attention. By focusing on your blood glucose management one day at a time, hopefully you will be able to maintain the best possible diabetes management and reward yourself for your efforts.

While there is quite a bit of information in this book, many other books are available that can help you in your quest to learn more about the positive self-care behaviors (listed below) that can help you. You may find additional ADA books to help you in the Resources section, page 151.

1. **Healthy Eating**
2. **Being Active**
3. **Monitoring**
4. **Taking Medication**
5. **Problem Solving**
6. **Reducing Risks**
7. **Healthy Coping**

Remember that you are not alone in your journey. In addition to your family and friends, your diabetes care team is there to help. They will assist you in gaining knowledge about self-care behaviors, identifying your goals, and figuring out obstacles that stand in your way. Together, you can determine a path to find the quality of life that you are striving to achieve.

Resources

For more information on everything from healthy eating and being active to taking medication and healthy coping, see these great American Diabetes Association books.

American Diabetes Association. *Diabetes A to Z. 7th ed.* Alexandria, VA: American Diabetes Association, 2016

American Diabetes Association. *Your Type 2 Diabetes Action Plan.* Alexandria, VA: American Diabetes Association, 2015

Garnero T. *Your First Year with Diabetes. 2nd ed.* Alexandria, VA: American Diabetes Association, 2013

Hayes C. *The "I Hate to Exercise" Book for People with Diabetes. 3rd ed.* Alexandria, VA: American Diabetes Association, 2013

Kay AB, Nelson LB. *Yoga & Diabetes.* Alexandria, VA: American Diabetes Association, 2015

Napora JP. *Stress-Free Diabetes.* Alexandria, VA: American Diabetes Association, 2010

Ross TA, Geil PB. *What Do I Eat Now? 2nd ed.* Alexandria, VA: American Diabetes Association, 2015

Warshaw HS. *Diabetes Meal Planning Made Easy. 5th ed.* Alexandria, VA: American Diabetes Association, 2016

Index

blood glucose level. *See also* self-
    monitoring blood glucose (SMBG)
  after-meal value, 34
  bedtime check, 34
  carbohydrate, 80, 122
  complication, 44
  excursions, 124
  exercise, 69
  fasting recommendation, 7
  medication interaction, 38
  middle of night check, 34–35
  monitoring, 7–8, 17–19, 33–36, 52, 54,
    70–71, 85–87, 102–103, 120–122,
    132, 134–135
  pattern, 36, 85–87, 102, 120
  pre-meal check, 34
  preventive care, 9–10
  recommended, 22, 24-26
  sick day management, 56
  travel, 135–136
  troubleshooting, 120–122
blood pressure, v, 7, 10, 24–25, 38, 43–44,
    60, 93, 126
blood vessel disease, 7, 10, 50, 59–60, 83,
    91
body mass index (BMI), 91
bone mineral density, 83
Borg Rate of Perceived Exertion (RPE),
    52–53
buffet, 117–118

C

calorie, 16, 49–50, 66, 80–82, 98, 100, 133
CalorieKing, 82, 115
carbohydrate
  blood glucose management, 80, 122
  Create Your Plate, 81
  eating out, 117
  exercise, 17
  fat-free food, 100
  free food, 99
  glucose source, 41
  healthy eating, 30–31
  hypoglycemia, 38
  medical nutrition therapy, 52
  portion size, 66

serving size, 51
sick day management, 57
tracking and recording, 15
type 2 diabetes, 2
cataract, 74
chair exercise, 101
childbirth, 2. *See also* pregnancy
children, vii, 39
cholesterol, v, 3, 7, 10, 25–26, 42–44, 50,
    60, 99
Choose My Plate, 82
chronic stressor, 62
clinical depression, 94
clothing, 32
complication
  blood glucose level, 44
  exercise, 16, 52
  hyperglycemia, 22
  lab values, 25
  medication, 19
  preventive care, vii, 89
  risk reduction, 9–10, 59, 124–125,
    140–144
  type 2 diabetes, 2
concentration, 95
congestive heart failure, 59
contrast dye, 93
coping
  depression, 94–95
  empowerment, 44–46
  living well with diabetes, 26–27
  mental health professional, 111–112
  self-care behavior, 10
  stressors, 61–63
  stress reduction, 76–78
  support group, 144–145
  taking charge, 127–128
coronary artery disease, 59
Create Your Plate, 81

D

DASH (Dietary Approaches to Stop
    Hypertension), 126
dehydration, 23–24
dental exam, 91
depression, 94–95, 111–112
desire, 11

portion size, 50, 52, 66–69, 82, 116–117
positive skills, 47–63
potassium, 126
prediabetes, vii, 2
pregnancy, 39, 142
prepregnancy counseling, 142
prescription, 37, 137, 139
preventive care, 59–60, 89–92, 140–144
Prevnar vaccine, 141–142
problem solving, 8–9
    blood glucose excursions, 124
    hyperglycemia, 22–24
    hypoglycemia, 39–42
    plan, 105–106
    preventive care, 89–92
    safety, 138–140
    self-management education, 72–74
    sick day management, 56–59
proliferative retinopathy, 74–75
prostaglandin suppository, 144
protected health information (PHI), 21
protein, 51–52

R
recordkeeping
    blood glucose level, 35–36, 124
    blood glucose pattern, 85–87, 90,
        102–103
    exercise pattern, 69
    foods eaten, 14–16
    medication, 19–21, 54
    self-management, 126
    stressors, 62
    trends and patterns, 12
red blood cell, 92
registered dietitian (RD), 15–16, 29, 42,
    50–52, 67, 82, 90, 93, 115
registered dietitian nutritionist (RDN),
    15–16, 29, 42, 50–52, 67, 82, 90, 93,
    115
reinforcement, 11–12
relaxation technique, 76
renal disease, 92. *See also* kidney disease
resilience, 26–27
resistance training, 7, 42, 83–85
respiratory tract infection, 24, 38
restaurant. *See* eating out

retina, 75
retinopathy, 75
reward system, 119, 148
risk reduction
    complication, 9–10, 140–144
    eye disease, 74–76
    kidney disease, 92–94
    nerve disease, 106–111
    self-care skills, 124–127
    target numbers, 22–24, 42–44
Round Health, 123

S
sadness, 95
safety, 138–140
salad dressing, 100, 117
saturated fat, 50, 60, 99
self-care behavior, 4–10, 27, 55, 78,
    124–128, 148. *See also* behavior
    modification
self-management, 29–47, 63, 97,
    126–127
self-management education, 24, 72–74,
    127
self-monitoring blood glucose (SMBG),
    7–8, 17–19, 33–36, 54, 85–87, 103,
    125
sensorimotor neuropathy, 106
serving size, 49–50. *See also* portion size
sexual dysfunction, 143–144
sharps, 88–89
shoe, 32, 52, 101, 107, 109–110, 135
sick day management, 9, 56–59, 105–106
sitting, 101–102
skill, 11
sleep, 95
SMART (Specific, Measurable,
    Achievable, Realistic, and
    Timebound), 45–46, 118
smartphone, 31, 72, 80, 82, 115, 123, 131
smoking, 91–92
snack, 31, 67, 116, 136, 138, 140
social activity, 32
social media, 145
sock, 32, 52, 109–110, 135
sodium, 51, 126
soybean oil, 100

statin, 25–26, 60
step, 32–33
Step Out: Walk to Stop Diabetes, 120
stimulation, 11
stress, 10, 61–63, 76–78, 94, 111, 125
stretch, 32, 83
stroke, 10, 59–60
sugar, 51
sugar alcohol, 99
suicide, 95
SuperTracker, 82
support system, 3–4, 26, 47, 119, 144–145

T
talk test, 52–53
Tdap vaccine, 142
teeth, 91
test strip, 17–18, 33, 54
time zone, 136
titration, 38
tobacco, 93. *See also* smoking
trans fat, 50, 60, 99
transplant, 93
trauma, 24
travel, 88–89, 135–138
triglyceride, 3, 7, 10, 60
TSA (Transportation Security
     Administration), 136–139
TuDiabetes.org, 145
tuning fork, 109
Twitter, 145

type 1 diabetes, 17
type 2 diabetes, vii, 2–3

U
United States Department of Agriculture
     (USDA), 82
United States Healthful Food Council, 114
urgent response system, 131
urinary protein, 43

V
vaccination, 140–142
vascular disease, 3
vegetable, 50, 68, 126
Verified Internet Pharmacy Practice Site
     (VIPPS), 105
VIPPS Seal, 105
vision, 74–75

W
walk, 32–33, 52, 73, 101, 120
weight loss, 82, 91
weight management, 7, 66
weight resistance training, 7, 84, 119, 133
whole grain, 50, 117

X
x-ray, 93

Z
Zoster vaccine, 142